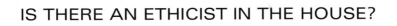
IS THERE AN ETHICIST IN THE HOUSE?

Bioethics and the Humanities

Eric M. Meslin and Richard B. Miller, editors

JONATHAN D. MORENO

IS THERE AN ETHICIST IN THE HOUSE?

ON THE CUTTING EDGE OF BIOETHICS

Indiana University Press

BLOOMINGTON AND INDIANAPOLIS

This book is a publication of

Indiana University Press
601 North Morton Street
Bloomington, IN 47404-3797 USA

http://iupress.indiana.edu

Telephone orders   800-842-6796
Fax orders   812-855-7931
Orders by e-mail   iuporder@indiana.edu

The paper used in this publication meets the
minimum requirements of American National
Standard for Information Sciences—Permanence of
Paper for Printed Library Materials, ANSI Z39.48-
1984.

Manufactured in the United States of America

Library of Congress Cataloging-in-Publication Data

Moreno, Jonathan D.
  Is there an ethicist in the house? : on the cutting edge
of bioethics. / Jonathan D. Moreno.
      p. ; cm. — (Bioethics and the humanities)
   Includes bibliographical references and index.
   ISBN 0-253-34635-5 (cloth : alk. paper)
   1. Medical ethics. 2. Bioethics.
   [DNLM: 1. Bioethical Issues—Collected Works.
2. Bioethics—Collected Works.] I. Title. II. Series.
   R724.M833 2005
   174.2—dc22
                                          2005001676

1 2 3 4 5 10 09 08 07 06 05

For Leslye, Jarrett, and Jillian

"Grief can take care of itself, but to get the full value
of joy you must have somebody to divide it with."
—Mark Twain

For in the end we are entirely dependent upon the universe,
and into sacrifices and surrenders of some sort,
deliberately looked at and accepted,
we are drawn and pressed,
as into our only permanent positions
of repose.

—William James

Contents

Introduction: "Is There a Philosopher in the House?"

"Is there a doctor in the house?" Often uttered in alarm, even panic, this cry for help locates the special expectations we hold for physicians: that they can bring much-needed expertise in dire circumstances, and that this expertise is to some degree a public resource to be shared without reservation, at least in an emergency.

By contrast, "Is there philosopher in the house?" might well serve as the gag line in a Woody Allen film—not because philosophers may not be of service in matters of practical intelligence (after twenty-five years in medical education I believe more firmly than ever that we are), but because there is rarely an urgent need for our services. Some would argue that urgency is, in fact, inherently contraindicated as a condition for philosophical reflection.

Consider, by contrast, "Is there an ethicist in the house?" Though I have not heard this phrase verbatim, I have heard its spirit expressed on any number of occasions, usually with an edge of anxiety. A nice question, one I take up early in this book, is what exactly is being asked for at such times. Whatever else is going on, the notion that the "ethicist" can bring some expertise to bear on the situation is presupposed in the encounters that stem from this professional role. The word *ethicist* has somehow come to connote a highly practical form of philosophical expertise, at times even crowding out the great range of philosophical inquiry with a less immediate focus. Thus, I was startled to hear Spinoza described on National Public Radio as an "ethicist," a term to which contemporary ears can relate but that tends to flatten out the metaphysical foundations of Spinoza's philosophy.

More generally, since ethics has taken an "applied" turn over the last several decades, it is best not to use moral philosophy as a synonym. In many quarters the study of ethics has come to be a multidisciplinary affair in which practitioners are expected to have at their command at least some knowledge of relevant legal, economic, political, social scientific, and often historical aspects of the topic. In the realm of professional ethics, deeper and more sustained reflection on moral philosophy, while always welcome, is generally not required. In other words, it has come to be perfectly respectable in the world of professional ethics (though scandalous to many philosophers), to draw upon philosophical resources without spending a lot of time enriching or expanding them.

In fact, as a graduate student in philosophy I took no ethics course, though I did pass a comprehensive exam for which I read, among other classics, Spencer's *Ethics,* often said to have set the tone for modern analytic moral philosophy. Spencer impressed me but left me cold. As excited as I was about the philosophy of science and the philosophy of language, even for a time about existential phenomenology, I could not work up a personal enthusiasm for moral theory. Kant's epistemology was endlessly fascinating and managed to be simultaneously rational and mysterious, but his ethics was clear, sensible, and led to an intellectual dead end.

Perhaps I was guilty of a failure of imagination partly due to juvenile certainty about the way the world ought to be, fed by an element of moral superiority in the late 1960s youth movement of which I was a part. I was not alone, of course, in finding ethics a vast wasteland. Much of my generation saw little point in worrying about moral theory when other young Americans and Vietnamese peasants of all ages were being killed and maimed without any sound explanation. As the country was being torn apart by an actual moral crisis, analytic philosophy seemed to offer at best a witty parlor game.

Yet the first philosophy course I took in college, the one that persuaded me to major in the subject, was ethics. My college professor, the late Evelyn Urban Shirk, was a product of Columbia's strongly naturalistic tradition and the author of a volume propounding what she called "ethical contextualism." Hers was a case-oriented approach that was decidedly short on theory, except the Deweyan sort that explained why theory didn't matter, or philosophy got theory wrong, or both. Evidently, I found this style very attractive. Several years later I encountered Dewey again in a graduate seminar with John J. McDermott, then at the City University of New York. Both Shirk and McDermott became friends and mentors, and they turned me toward a lifetime of identification with the classical American philosophers—especially John Dewey, William James, and Charles S. Peirce. But I couldn't see a reason to place ethics in the forefront of my intellectual agenda. Instead, as a student of the philosopher of science Richard Rudner at Washington University in St. Louis, I wrote a doctoral dissertation in which I pursued themes from the early pragmatists that persisted in the writing of Nelson Goodman and Willard Quine.

Following graduate school, a series of fortuitous events led me toward bioethics while still bypassing any hint of interest in ethical theory. In New York I had struck up a friendship with Art Caplan that continued while we finished our graduate work. I followed his sojourn at the Hastings Center with mild interest, visiting him there once long enough to play volleyball with the staff. The year was 1978, and though the pace of bioethics was picking up, the Center seemed a languorous place, though only because I had not yet witnessed the grant-writing process.

A year later I started work in the philosophy department at George Washington University. There was a need for a philosopher in a new, experimental course on bioethics with students and faculty from throughout the university. As an untenured junior professor looking for ways to make myself invaluable to the department, I eagerly signed on, fortunate to be teamed with Gail Povar, then a young physician who taught me the medical ropes while I stayed one step ahead of the class in the ethics readings. Beginning with Gail, I have been fortunate to have had a long line of physician colleagues who taught me most of what I know about clinical ethics. With them in mind, I try to recall daily that, whatever philosophers may opine, it is doctors, nurses, and their patients who bear the immediate burden of the latest moral nostrum.

As Hegel would have it, quantity changed to quality as bioethics assumed a growing place in my consciousness. I wondered what advice Dewey would give to a young philosopher in the last twenty years of the twentieth century, had he the opportunity to do so. "Go bioethics, young man," seemed a likely response. I did so, taking a position at the Hastings Center in 1984 and returning to George Washington a year later with a joint appointment in the medical school, then downstate to SUNY and a full-time job as a professor of bioethics in 1988. A ten-year early-career transition was complete. In the ensuing years, first in Washington and New York and then at the University of Virginia, I undertook the work that is represented in these essays.

My early interest in the history of American philosophy, and of the work of Dewey and William James in particular, turned out to be an intellectual framework that I carried with me into bioethics. With its emphasis on the lived experience and on the notion that moral values emerge from that experience, I have long thought that only a lack of familiarity with American philosophical naturalism has caused bioethicists to ignore this very suitable framework for the broad range of activities included in bioethical practice. Eric Meslin once suggested to me that I am one of a very few writers in bioethics with a "philosophical program," a reference to the development of a conceptual framework and its application to a range of problems. He had a point. My naturalism is on display in various ways in this volume: reference to my own personal and professional experience, a case-oriented approach, and an emphasis on historical inquiry in making sense of current circumstances and judgments.

In the twenty-five years since I entered the field, the literature in bioethics has undergone explosive growth, with many very talented and insightful writers. As the bioethics field has matured, it has also undergone inevitable specialization. The subjects I address in this book represent the areas in which I think I have made the most original contribution, especially bioethical naturalism, human research ethics, and national security experiments. In all of these cases, I have tried to elaborate rich bioethical possibilities that I believe have been insufficiently noted. This volume is therefore not an introduction to bioethics so much as a re-visioning of the field from a certain angle, one that I can only hope is more acute than obtuse.

List of Abbreviations

ACHRE	Advisory Committee on Human Radiation Experiments
ADAMHA	Agency for Drug Addiction and Mental Health Association
AFMPC	Armed Forces Medical Policy Council
ASHG	American Society for Human Genetics
CMR	Committee on Medical Research
DHEW	Department of Health, Education, and Welfare
DHHS	Department of Health and Human Services
DOD	Department of Defense
IRB	institutional review board
NBAC	National Bioethics Advisory Commission
NIH	National Institutes of Health
NIMH	National Institute of Mental Health

PART ONE

A HOSPITAL PHILOSOPHER

Once during a break in a Hastings Center research group meeting while I was on the staff, the subject of informal conversation was how those at the table got interested in bioethics. I don't remember how the subject arose, but it turned out that most group members, which included guests at the meeting as well as center associates, could cite a specific experience, often a highly personal one that clearly turned them in this direction. I'm sure I learned more about these people from that brief exchange than from all the hours we sat at the table working on the project.

Ever since then I have thought that bioethics is a personal subject in a way that other professional ethics fields are not. After all, as children we all have encounters with nurses and physicians, but not with lawyers or engineers. I have often started classes with first-year medical students by asking them to recall their early encounters with doctors. Often these were very important to their decision to go to medical school, but not always because they had happy memories.

I have always believed that there is no interesting gap between bioethics, especially in the clinical setting, and narrative, and therefore I have been quite comfortable with the narrative and case-based approach to bioethics. The first part of the book is thus unavoidably somewhat autobiographical as I attempt in various ways to articulate my experience doing ethics in the clinical setting. That experience took place largely between 1986 and 1997 at George Washington University, Children's Hospital in Washington, and the SUNY Health Science Center at Brooklyn and several of its affiliates. In that period I encountered several kinds of cases that continue to strike me as illustrating paradigmatic problems for the "hospital philosopher." These cases provide illustrations of the clinical ethics consensus that has developed since I entered the field.

> *A man in his late 60s has end-stage kidney disease. He is hospitalized because his condition cannot be controlled with medication. He also has a history of alcoholism and has wandered around the region for years doing odd jobs. He has no contact with his family. Long-term dialysis is recommended, but he refuses, saying he doesn't want "to live that way." When examined, he is alert and knows that he is in the hospital, but his mental status exam suggests that he could have dementia.*

The fact that this man is socially alienated is no reason to value his life differently from that of anyone else's. Therefore strenuous attempts must be made both to identify the extent and character of his dementia, if any, and to ascertain his authentic preferences. Like many of us who first face serious disease, he may at first underestimate his true wish to continue living and overestimate the burden of dialysis. The undeniable costs to society of his continuing care are not to be considered on an ad hoc basis by his doctors and nurses; these are political questions that in a democracy must be addressed by the electorate.

> *An elderly woman with severe emphysema collapsed at home and was brought to hospital by ambulance, where she was resuscitated. She has been put on a respirator because she cannot breathe on her own, but now her physician is not able to wean her from the machine. She communicates competently with hand signals and writes notes in complete sentences. After several weeks she*

writes, "Take me off this thing. I want to die. I've had enough. I didn't want to be brought back to live on a machine in the first place."

As in the previous case, self-determination is the presumptive first principle in our society for this mature adult. One is not required to accept medical treatment against one's competent will. However, her apparent capacity to decide might be complicated by depression, which is common in older persons, and this should be ruled out. If a thorough medical assessment concludes that she faces ventilator dependence for an uncertain period, and if she is found capable of making this particular irreversible decision, the burden will fall on the argument that she should be kept on a machine against her will. Finally, other medical complications are likely to intervene, but the decision to withdraw, perhaps after a trial of antidepressants, cannot be long delayed.

A 16-year-old boy has been unconscious for several months after an automobile accident. He breathes independently but is fed through a stomach tube. The doctors have told his parents that his outlook is not good, that at best he will suffer from brain damage if he does finally wake up. His mother feels that her son is some-how suffering, and she can't bear to see him in the hospital. She thinks it would be best for him and for the family if they let him go, which she thinks is God's will. Her husband disagrees. He wants to press on under any circumstances and holds out hope that the doctors are wrong about his son's prospects.

Few circumstances are more agonizing for families and for the medical team than a child's severe illness accompanied by dis-agreement between parents. This young man has evidently had no opportunity to express, or even to develop, his own values and preferences about his treatment should he ever be in this tragic situation. Therefore his best interests are to guide decision mak-ing for him, though his parents seem to disagree about what those interests are. Prognostication for a younger person who has been unconscious for this amount of time is difficult, but in general it is thought better to err on the side of life unless and until the medical and scientific consensus would hold that the underlying neural systems required for awareness have been hopelessly compromised. At that point it is hard to see what interest he would have in continued vegetative existence. Perhaps most critical at the early stage, however, is an intervention that would help his parents develop an integrated and mutually supporting relationship for the sake of their son's ultimate welfare.

These are, of course, life and death cases. As such they are not necessarily representative of the less dramatic but also consequential problems that face clinical ethicists. However, the fact remains that these are the kinds of cases that first attract most people to bioethics, and because there is a special gravity to decisions about mortality, they present an especially sharp challenge to our values. Though these tests cannot be avoided, neither should we ever be confident that we have settled them once and for all.

1

Is There an Ethicist in the House?

HERR PROFESSOR DR.

Some years ago, a *New Yorker* cartoon depicted a stuffy maitre d'
on the telephone at the reception podium of an obviously fancy
restaurant. "Yes, Dr. Adams," he said. "That will be two for dinner at seven. Now, is that an actual M.D. or only a Ph.D.?"

As a philosopher who teaches in a medical school, this cartoon
has special meaning for me. Like many others, I have long wondered about the business of using academic titles as part of one's
name. Is the use of "Dr." a mark of arrogance, or is its omission
self-denial and nondisclosure? The most prestigious college I was
associated with before I turned away from traditional philosophy
teaching identified all its instructors as "Mr." or "Ms." in the
course list. But I also recall my senior colleague in another philosophy department who invariably introduced himself, with a
broad smile and hearty handshake, as "Professor" so-and-so. I remember thinking that he said it as though that was his first name.

I started out in bioethics by team teaching in medical school
courses offered in the medical school building. I noticed that my

medical colleagues would usually introduce me to the students as "Dr. Moreno." It was apparent that everyone was comfortable with this mode of address, or at least not uncomfortable, including the philosophy majors taking the course for philosophy credit who knew me as "Professor Moreno" elsewhere on the campus. The physical location of the course supported the "Dr." emphasis, including the meeting room itself, which was a lab suitably arrayed with cabinets, beakers, Bunsen burners, and emergency showerheads.

Under these circumstances it would have been pointless to note that the title indicating degree is less prestigious than that indicating rank. First, my rank wasn't really professor at that time—where's the prestige in being an assistant professor?—and second, the marks of status in the German academic tradition don't apply in the New World, where even generic "doctors" have at least as much clout as generic "professors." My dissertation director once recalled his work for a think tank on contract with the navy. When operational issues came up, the brass said, "Let's call the doctors." "Let's call the professors" wouldn't have been believable enough on its face to be a cute inside joke. A medical school administrator with a doctorate in another humanities field told me that he permits himself to be called "Dr." within the institution, since otherwise he would not be taken seriously by the medical and science faculty, though he would loathe to be so addressed in any other context.

When still shuttling between a liberal arts college and medical school, I was also able to adapt any doubts I had about the propriety of being titled one way or another to the context. This adjustment worked well until my first summer on rounds in an oncology unit. Joining the team for its tours of the bedside was an opportunity to learn more about the physicians' work style. With this experience I could formulate more relevant suggestions when we gathered around the conference table to discuss their more difficult cases.

Upon entering a patient's room I would be introduced by the attending physician as one of the many doctors on the team. Indeed, on morning rounds there were ordinarily eight or ten of us huddled around a bed, several of whom were no more medical doctors—indeed, less "doctors"—than me, but were medical students or pharmacists. The attending oncologist was invariably polite to the patient, but rather than running through the whole list of people assembled, would often simply say something like, "These are some of the doctors who are on the team caring for you."

Since truth-telling was supposed to be a matter for my watch, the experience was unsettling, though my colleague, the attending physician, assured me that I had every right to be part of the team and to be introduced in a like fashion. In one sense I could hardly argue, since the psychologists were also undifferentiated as "doctors" and had the appropriate degrees. My stumbling block was the knowledge that none of these people would have expected a philosopher to be among those privileged to witness their vulnerability, so how could I presume their acquiescence?

Though it was not the primary reason I was drawn to spend more clinical time in the neonatal intensive care unit, the title issue is less of a problem with those tiny patients. In the NICU it is easy for the attending neonatologist to introduce me as "Dr. Moreno, our medical ethicist" to the staff without raising eyebrows. Sapient patients, on the other hand, might well wonder why such a presence is needed.

TEACHING ETHICS, DOING SOCIOLOGY

Whatever sensitivity I brought to these matters can be attributed partly to my close association with Barry Glassner and his colleagues who founded the *Journal of Qualitative Sociology* in the late 1970s. At that time, fresh out of graduate school, I could not have anticipated my bioethical turn. I enjoyed reading the manuscripts submitted to *QS* and attending sociology conferences—the issues were delightfully different from those that drove my philosophical colleagues—but I had no idea that this way of thinking would ever have direct relevance to my working life.

About ten years after my initial experience with qualitative sociology, I conducted a weekly ethics seminar with pediatric nurses. They were a marvelous group, smart and dedicated. The first several sessions were on various standard issues in medical ethics, and we then focused on the peculiar stresses inherent in the nurse's role. One of these is the need to deal with various attending physicians who have different practice styles and make very different demands on the staff. An important part of learning how to nurse in a particular unit is learning how to deal with the attendings. Some annoyance was expressed, but mostly resignation.

Then I suggested that the young residents, who are, after all, on wards a lot more than the attendings, must present another sort of challenge. I mentioned my impression that nurses don't deal with all these physicians-in-training in the same ways. This general remark immediately elicited smiles of recognition, some more bashful than others, and a few amused glances at one another. Emboldened, I then allowed that I have sometimes observed nurses "game" or manipulate the house staff to get what they want. Confirming anecdotes then poured forth freely, most on the order of knowing which resident to approach to deal with a problem and how to do so. An especially memorable conversation followed about nurses' relationships with female residents. For at least some of these nurses, those dealings were freighted with a great deal of complexity.

In retrospect, what I found especially fascinating about this discussion in the nursing ethics seminar was not the content of their stories about gaming the residents with whom they worked, but the zeal and amused delight with which some of them talked about it. The affect in the room differed considerably from our previous discussion of their relations with the attendings, for in that dynamic they were subordinate. When it came to the house staff, they were in a position of power by virtue of knowing more about how the institution worked than the newer residents. Of course the young doctors had to learn, said one, but it was hard to watch them learn on the patients that they were also charged with caring for, especially when the nurses had to clean up after their mistakes. On the whole, while they were not unsympathetic to the new doctors' plight, it was pleasurable for these experienced women who perceived themselves as often undervalued by the institution to exercise a little dominance over some of the supposedly best and brightest.

I was delighted with this session and with how much it had revealed about the interstices of the hospital regime. The nurses themselves also expressed their enjoyment at having a phenomenon framed for them, for although they were roughly aware of it, they had not fully articulated it before or talked about it with one another. In fact, the last minutes of that class were devoted to a heartfelt discussion about interpersonal honesty and authenticity, and about how hard this is to achieve in the highly scrutinized, hierarchical, and closely regulated modern hospital.

Talking openly about power and dominance is an agenda I have tried to pursue with residents themselves. Even though this is arguably not "medical ethics" in a strict academic sense, the constraints on healthcare workers' efforts to take good care of their patients obviously have moral overtones. I meet regularly with groups of residents in conferences in which ethical issues are given the stage. If these sessions are defined as "core curriculum" rather than "patient management," they enjoy the great advantage of having no attending physicians in the room, but only the house officers themselves. After a few meetings I am usually able to engender a level of trust that enables topics to be opened in the ethics conference that are not spoken of in any other formal setting. The most powerful of these sessions had to do with the saying that mistakes are dealt with in the department, a topic I was able to introduce by describing Charles Bosk's classic observations about a surgical residency program in *Forgive and Remember* (1979).

ALIENATED ALIENS

In the hospitals where I worked in Brooklyn, most of the residents in primary care departments are graduates of medical schools in other countries, usually foreign nationals on special visas. One might have thought that they would be less inclined to criticize systems of authority, especially as tenuous accredited guests, than are residents who are citizens and who are socialized and educated in American institutions. But in fact, I have found them remarkably willing to question their situation and, because of their cultural perspective, far sharper in their critiques of our system. On rare occasions they are deeply embittered. A Russian surgeon attempting to gain credentials to practice here denounced the American colleagues he had observed as motivated entirely by greed. At least in the old Soviet system, for all its faults, there was room for compassion, he concluded, and the treatment was actually better than what he had seen here. The others in his cohort, some also Russian and some from other parts of the world, were obviously taken aback by his caustic outburst and quickly asserted that his observations applied only to a minority of American physicians they had met.

Coming from such countries as the Philippines, Pakistan, and Argentina, these exceptionally capable people often have practiced medicine at home, have not set foot in the United States before, and within days of their arrival are at work in some of our busiest inner-city hospitals. They tend to be among the best products of their country's system of medical education, but they are viewed as second class in the United States, and they know it. Current federal policy changes call for a vast reduction in the number of positions available for "international medical graduates," who give most of the in-patient care in places like Brooklyn.

For some who have difficulty obtaining a visa in time to begin their residency, the indignities begin even before they arrive. For others the shock comes later: one young man arrived in this country in mid-June, days before his orientation, settled his family in a tough neighborhood near the hospital, and had his car stolen before he even began to work. He immediately moved his wife and children to suburban New Jersey and took the long commute several times a week.

The first time I met with a group of new arrivals, I realized that because they had no understanding of the American legal system and little familiarity with many of our cultural assumptions, they could hardly make sense of discussions of patient autonomy or informed consent. Sometimes their reactions to our system achieved comical proportions. One melodramatic chief resident told me facetiously that in his country "when one of my patients died the government sends me a letter—thanking me! Because there are too many people! Here, if one of my patients dies I get a letter from a lawyer!"

More usually what I have found in these sessions, which I think of as anthropologic focus groups, is amazement at our cultural contradictions. For example, one Latin American who had been a professor of histology in a medical school back home was non-plussed at Dr. Kevorkian's ability to "get away with murder" in public. In his country, he said, that would be impossible. When he was questioned, he admitted that assisted suicide probably does happen, but if a doctor did that in a publicized manner, he would certainly be imprisoned. The example enabled me to explain that our constitution gives the states authority to create their own laws on matters such as the regulation of healthcare professionals, and that at the time Kevorkian started, Michigan had no law on physician-assisted suicide.

Although the group was frankly puzzled by the moral inconsistencies of a society that rhetorically insists on the sanctity of human life, those from Catholic countries had to admit that the same was true of their homelands, where abortion is illegal but common. In the end, these young physicians are candid that they are not here for philosophical consistency but for professional training and economic opportunity. They are willing to accept American social conflicts as minefields they must be willing to navigate in order to reap personal rewards.

TAKE TWO LOGICAL CONNECTIVES AND CALL ME IN THE MORNING

Many of the venues in which I work are more or less academic rather than mainly clinical. They include conferences with residents in which issues in medical ethics are discussed as well as grand rounds about topics like euthanasia. These events are in many ways extensions of graduate and continuing education on philosophical and policy problems. When these academic exercises shade into finding solutions to clinical issues with ongoing cases, a new and different role for the philosopher, the most fascinating experiences I have had in the sociology of the professions are engendered. Requests for concrete advice about managing what the physicians involved perceive to be ethical problems are, of course, common and expected for one touted as the "ethicist." More often than not, the problem with a current case has to do with a concern or disagreement with a patient's family about the most appropriate course of treatment. Under these circumstances, negotiating skills are as important as philosophical insight.

Sometimes, however, requests for advice go beyond what can be viewed as ethical issues and into technical medical questions, such as what order and technique for the withdrawal of life-sustaining treatment should be adopted. Sometimes these questions do have ethical implications, since deciding to stop antibiotics for a dying patient is distinct from turning off a ventilator, though the end result is the same. On the other hand, I have also been asked how much sedation should be given when the respirator is being withdrawn (to prevent a feeling of suffocation), or at what rate the supply of oxygen should be reduced. These questions have been asked by physicians who are quite aware that I am not a medical doctor, but they ascribe to me a level of experience with technical matters by virtue of the clinical issues that animate my intellectual work.

Another reason for this exaggerated notion of the philosopher-ethicist's knowledge base is that some (but by no means all) ethicists have medical titles. When I worked at SUNY Downstate, my rank and tenure were in pediatrics, and I held a joint appointment in medicine as well. I am sure that my opinions would have been taken far less seriously if my professorship had been in philosophy, as it was at a previous institution, rather than in central clinical departments. The assumption was that I have somehow "earned my stripes" to have these appointments. While I would like to think that is true, contingent factors are also at work in the way that ethicists are assigned their academic titles.

These generalizations are, of course, severely limited, and in particular cases, attitudes toward the nonphysician presuming to speak to clinical issues vary widely. At one extreme, even close colleagues have sometimes trumped my arguments about physician paternalism by appealing to ad hominem tactics that I heard more frequently ten years ago than I do now: "Well it may look that way to a philosopher, but it's different for the physician who is actually giving the treatment." At another extreme, I have been appointed to ad hoc committees on sensitive administrative problems (such as what to do about a resident who was HIV positive but wanted to stay in the program), even though ethical expertise was not much needed. In such cases I have come to see myself as cast into the role of a "secular priest": even in a pluralistic and multiethnic society someone must sanctify such delicate proceedings. If responsible authorities can announce that the ethicist was part of the committee, then they are generally perceived to have taken into account something important, though it is not easy to say exactly what that is.

IS THERE A DOCTOR ON BOARD?

In spite of my frequent public professions that my goal is not to be a physician manqué but a philosopher of medicine, immersion in a medical environment and collaboration with medical professionals have deeply affected my self-identification. I was not aware of how much I have come to identify with the physician role until a long airplane flight several years ago. I was seated in a wide-body aircraft in a row on the side of the plane in front of an emergency exit and near the galley, the kind of seat in which there is an open space that permits even the economy traveler to stretch out. With no seats in front of me and the seat next to me unoccupied, I congratulated myself that on this flight I had first-class space for a lot less.

Several hours after dinner night descended, and I managed to drift off. Not long after, I felt something landing on top of my feet. It was a female passenger whom the flight attendants were attempting to place in a position where she could be examined. The cabin was darkened and the voices muffled by engine noise, but I gathered that the passenger had collapsed after leaving the toilet. The flight attendants hoped it was only airsickness, but they feared a heart attack. Quickly the call went out for a physician on board, and the first class cabin seemed to empty as an international group of medical personnel huddled over a shrouded figure below me.

All this happened in a few moments, of course, while I was semi-conscious, but I remember being struck by an urgent desire to answer the flight attendants' call for assistance and to join my "colleagues" at the "bedside." That I could contribute little or nothing to the ministrations being provided (which consisted mainly of a brief medical history, a self-report of symptoms, and the provision of some oxygen) had nothing to do with my reflex sense that I had a place with the "team." Since then I have had another such experience, and again I wanted to announce myself to the flight crew: "I'm not a medical doctor, but I am an ethicist. Can I be of assistance?" Fortunately for all concerned, I have resisted such urges and concentrated instead on the introspection for which my training more properly qualifies me.

On the other hand, maybe someday I will answer that call. . . .

2

Call Me Doctor?

Confessions of a Hospital Philosopher

AT THE BEDSIDE

I stood over the incubator as the neonatal fellow rattled off the list of known and suspected deformities: cleft palate, micro-penis, tetrology of Fallot (a complex of heart defects), misplaced liver and spleen, probably severe brain damage according to CT scan, all consistent with trisomy 13 (a genetic disease) but no definitive lab results so far. I glanced at the faces of the group assembled for rounds. The attending neonatologist chewed her lower lip pensively during the recital, staring at the baby. She was the only one about my age (38); the rest were at least five years younger. As one should expect of Brooklyn, the group was an ethnic smorgasbord: Central and South American, Caribbean, Asian, Jewish, African American, Pakistani. The baby in this case was Irish. The young parents and much of the extended family were expected to visit him in the Neonatal Intensive Care Unit shortly, perhaps to say goodbye.

I had first become involved with this case about a week before when the neonatologist called me to ask for a "formal consult." At that time the question was whether the parents should be advised to proceed with heart surgery, which would be only the first step of a very uncertain course, causing suffering for the baby who might already be dying. The surgeon was very critical but willing, the nursery team anxious but inclined to intervene. After a lengthy discussion, it was agreed that the parents should be given several more days to decide, while reassuring them that everyone in the unit stood ready to support their decision.

In the interim, more grim diagnostic information had become available about the condition of the infant's brain and gut. The parents decided not to consent to surgery. The ethical problem that followed was shockingly clear: with a hormone called prostaglandin artificially administered, the infant's heart would be functional for weeks or even months, but eventually he would die, either due to the ultimately dysfunctional heart or from another of many possible catastrophes. The neonatologist looked at me and posed the simple question, "Should I stop the prostaglandin?"

It was the kind of moment those who conduct regular clinical ethics rounds both live for and dread. On one hand, whatever experience I have gained and intellectual subtlety I possess were being put to a poignant test; on the other hand, any qualification in my position could easily be viewed as evasive and might further frustrate the neonatal team. My Socratic reflexes took over: "What is the role of the prostaglandin absent the possibility of benefit from surgery?" Through a series of tortured questions and answers, I suggested that the central issue was this: Under the circumstances, was the hormone lifesaving or death-prolonging?

When I left the unit a few minutes later, I glanced at the baby boy's parents, grandparents, and an aunt and uncle, circled around him. His mother lifted him uncertainly out of his tiny bed, wondering, I supposed, if this would be the last time she held him.

Pushing open the double doors from the university hospital to the building that houses our medical center's offices, laboratories, and classrooms, I had a moment of vertigo. While it is true that many physicians still resist a role for philosophers in the clinical setting, the fact is that no one is "trained" for this. In helping to prevent needless suffering, was I making things too easy for everyone? But how could any of this be called easy? I thought about my own little boy and my then-unborn daughter: if, God forbid, one of them became terribly ill, would I want someone like me helping to make the decision about when to let them die? No one is "trained" for this, I repeated to myself.

ENTER THE PHILOSOPHERS

There is no accurate count of the number of academically credentialed philosophers who regularly consult in the clinical setting, but considering that it can't be more than a couple of hundred, they have received disproportionate attention from the public and the medical and nursing professions. Other philosophers, working in more traditional settings, have given this phenomenon a reception ranging from the contemptuous to the enthusiastic. Physician-ethicists are often seen by their medical colleagues as disconnected from their professional roots or downright intrusive, while lawyer-ethicists are often thought of in terms of the traditional rubric of the hospital attorney. With their education in moral philosophy, logic, and epistemology, the philosophers should in one sense be natural candidates for this kind of work. There is no surprise in the fact that the philosophers' reception among physicians has run along a broad spectrum, a matter to which I shall return.

Along with seminars in moral theory, many graduate students in philosophy are now learning specifically about medical ethics, and some are even gaining clinical experience before they receive their degrees, though this is a very small group. My own case was more typical of those who entered bioethics in the 1970s. I completed a dissertation on the history of American philosophy of language and set out for a traditional academic career. With a great deal of help from some mentors and a little luck in a brutal job market, six years after graduating I was more or less established in the profession. I was able to satisfy my burning desire to teach the subject I love, never having imagined that I might someday find the classroom limiting, and occasionally I wrote or delivered an arcane paper in which I took pride.

Yet after only a few years I grew uneasy. The thinkers who had most fascinated me in college and graduate school were those who found themselves at the intersection of great ideas and great public events: Socrates before the Athenian jury, Spinoza ostracized by the Dutch community, Dewey leading the liberal charge. It was John Dewey's career and his conception of values as natural features of experience that I found especially compelling. But unlike Dewey, I gradually realized, I lived in a time when intellectuals had effectively become marginalized in American society. As Russell Jacoby (1987) has pointed out, the academy is now virtually the only environment that will host intellectuals in America, or perhaps the only one they are prepared to inhabit. In spite of my genuine interest in certain technical questions in philosophy, I had a still greater wish to be a "public philosopher" in the Deweyan mold, but brought up to date.

I don't know if many of my colleagues among the "hospital philosophers" had a similar motivation, but I suspect some of them did. As a role in a multidisciplinary bioethics course at George Washington University became a regular part of my teaching load, the idea occurred to me that bioethics could provide the venue I sought. I also had observed the careers of two friends, first Art Caplan, now at the University of Pennsylvania, and then Larry McCullough, now at Baylor College of Medicine. Both had taken the direct route to bioethics following their philosophy Ph.D.s, and both soon became prominent in the field.

While teaching in the bioethics course, I became aware of another angle on my interest, some personal experiences that I had managed not to reflect upon very much. When I was five years old my mother underwent a radical amputation of her right arm and shoulder. Just before metastatic disease would have affected her vital organs, following months of wandering around the world in search of an answer to the riddle of the growing, painful egg-shaped lump in her upper arm, a rare chondorosarcoma was diagnosed. In the following years that period acquired a nearly mythical status in our house. I grew up with tales of the incompetent physicians, those who were kind but mystified, those who were contemptuous of another hysterical female patient, the young internist who finally solved the puzzle, and the gifted surgeon. I heard too about the German masseuse who swore she had never seen a supposed arthritis manifest itself this way. How all this affected me psychologically I cannot say; I only remember standing hesitantly at the far side of the living room when my mother returned from the hospital, worried that I would see blood.

Seventeen years later my 85-year-old father, a distinguished psychiatrist, collapsed during an influenza epidemic in which he suffered a severe case of flu. He had already suffered a series of tiny strokes, and his condition rapidly deteriorated. He announced his dying by refusing to eat. My parents had a pact that they would permit the other to die at home, but shortly after he began to fast, my father became incoherent and asked to be taken to the hospital. While most of his students and colleagues had been supportive of our actions, one of his close collaborators, also a psychiatrist, expressed grave distress to me that we were not intervening aggressively. Making a critical decision, my mother decided that pain was clouding his judgment and that this was his way of begging for relief from the suffering. At that point his personal physician agreed to give him massive doses of morphine. He died peacefully, in his own room, a few weeks later.

I now realize that the atmosphere surrounding my childhood since my mother's amputation was one in which certain ideas about the medical profession were henceforth taken for granted: that there was nothing magical about medicine, that fools coexisted with physicians of extraordinary ability, and that there was often no easy way to tell them apart. Most of all I came to understand that technique without judgment is insufficient in the make-up of a healer. But then, as though to forestall arrogance about this insight, when my father began his last illness I came to appreciate how elusive wisdom can be.

FROM PHILOSOPHY TO BIOETHICS

The public image of the bioethicist, such as it is, has diversified in the past decade. Not only is the bioethics expert a social critic, commenting on the role of biomedicine in human affairs in the large sense, but he or she may also—or even exclusively—take the role of clinical consultant at the bedside. As a philosopher, it is my newly found place in the clinical setting that most distinguishes me from my tradition.

This encounter with sickness is extraordinarily challenging for one whose primary professional identification is that of philosopher, for the intellectual detachment usually associated with philosophical speculation is at least as difficult to sustain in the oncology unit, for example, and may even seem voyeuristic. At the same time, before the current generation no cadre of philosophers had been permitted to become immersed so intimately in the health-care workers' struggles with suffering; indeed, in many instances we have been fairly dragged into the fray by beleaguered doctors. The new alliance between medicine and philosophy is particularly striking in light of the historic ambivalence in the relationship. The cult of Hippocrates was a mystical rather than a philosophical school, and Plato's Socrates frequently expressed skepticism about the usefulness of a call on the physician. Yet tradition has it that, just before his death, Socrates asked that one of his students give an offering to Aesculapius, the god of healing arts.

I have become preoccupied with two questions that emerge from this novel relationship between philosophy and medicine: First, does this experience, fascinating as it may be on other counts, have anything to contribute to the ancient line of philosophical inquiry per se? And second, what exactly is the philosopher qua philosopher contributing at the bedside?

Obviously these are interlocking questions. One asks what the Western philosophical tradition, understood in the usual way as originating with Socrates and Plato and manifesting itself variously in such twentieth-century movements as logical positivism, pragmatism, and phenomenology, have to gain from the experiences of philosophers in medical centers. The other asks what philosophers in medical centers have to give back to the patients and professionals they are privileged to encounter.

Of course, in the most general sense, the fact of mortality has an honored place in Western philosophy, exemplified classically in Socrates' aphorism about philosophy as training for death. However, it is not mortality that I am referring to here so much as morbidity, illness that may be acute or chronic, terminal or temporary. By contrast with the impression that the reality of death has made on philosophers, there are fewer well-known examples of the contributions that observations of morbidity, of disease whether or not terminal, have made upon philosophers. One of these few was left us by William James, who worked in a German insane asylum while on leave from medical school recuperating from his own breakdown. James one day came upon an epileptic patient,

> a black haired youth with greenish skin, entirely idiotic, who used to sit all day on one of the benches, or rather shelves against the wall, which his knees drawn up against his chin, and the coarse gray undershirt, which was his only garment, drawn up over them inclosing his entire figure. This image and my fear entered into a species of combination with each other. That shape am I, I felt potentially. Nothing that I possess can defend me against that fate, if the hour for it should strike for me as it struck for him. . . . After this the universe was changed forever. (1968, 6)

In fact, James must have exaggerated the suddenness of this existential insight, for he had already experienced illness and depression (covered under the nineteenth-century rubric of "neurasthenia") both in his brilliant sister Alice and in himself. (His brother Henry seemed in control of the disorder but not unaffected.) But the contemplation of this helpless young man was apparently an epiphany for James, crystallizing the key proposition of his young life: to take the initiative by willing his own freedom, to exercise what he would later call the will to believe. "Not in maxims, not in *Anschauungen,* but in accumulated *acts* of thought lies salvation. . . . My belief, to be sure, *can't* be optimistic—but I will posit life (the real, the good) in the self-governing *resistance* of the ego to the world. Life shall be built in doing and suffering and creating" (1968, 8).

James's observation of mental illness from "outside" as a clinician and as a sibling, combined with his experiences "inside" his own depression, led him down a certain philosophic path. The French philosopher Renouvier's pluralistic antideterminism was a first step, then maturing into a vision of a "pluriverse" of open possibilities rather than a priori fixities. For James, the ever-present possibility of disease, and especially of our supposed inability to thwart our personal destiny, helped open a set of philosophical possibilities.

To finish this short story about the way the experience of disease has worked its way at least into Anglo-American philosophy, I want to indicate its influence upon James's successor, John Dewey. "Suffering" in James's language carries more than a hint of ambiguity, referring not only to the misery associated with specific states (as is typically the case when suffering is accompanied by physical pain or mental anguish) but also to the more general sense in which life is constantly marked by "suffering" in the sense of the subject of external influences. It is this latter, broader sense of suffering that Dewey regards, along with "doing," as one of the two defining moments of experience. Indeed, according to Dewey's naturalistic metaphysics intelligent doing would be impossible without suffering, for there would be no leads concerning what to act upon, or how or when to do so. In Dewey's philosophical anthropology, suffering is elevated to the level of a generic trait of existence: in a literal sense, we are all patients.

Hence, we are all subject to the precarious nature of existence. Dewey's recitation of the anthropological data on the universal awareness of this brute fact is sharp and undeniable, worth citing at length from his 1929 work, *Experience and Nature:*

> Man finds himself living in an aleatory world; his existence involves, to put it badly, a gamble. The world is a scene of risk; it is uncertain, unstable, uncannily unstable. Its dangers are irregular, inconstant, not to be counted upon as to their times and seasons. Although persistent, they are sporadic, episodic. It is darkest just before dawn; pride goes before a fall; the moment of greatest prosperity is the moment most charged with ill-omen, most opportune for the evil eye. Plague, famine, failure of crops, disease, death, defeat in battle, are always just around the corner, and so are abundance, strength, victory, festival, and song. Luck is proverbially both good and bad in its distributions. The sacred and the accursed are potentialities of the same situation; and there is no category of things which has not embodied the sacred and the accursed: persons, words, places, times, directions in space, stones, winds, animals, stars. (1958, 41)

This passage is perhaps striking enough for the fact that its author is not usually regarded as a philosopher driven by dark passions; it gains still more meaning and poignancy with the knowledge that Dewey had by this time experienced the deaths of two of his children.

My point has been to give an example of the way philosophical reflection can, in a dramatic and substantive way, be influenced by illness as a feature of human life. But this story about James and Dewey is not necessarily illustrative of the ways that the contemporary philosopher, in the role of philosopher, may gather grist from regular attendance in a hospital. That opportunity presented itself in the past few years as a result of an unprecedented confluence of circumstances in the delivery of health care. These circumstances include the familiar technological breakthroughs that permit the extension of life but not its return to its previous quality as well as less-elevated concerns, especially the pervasive fear of suit among physicians. It is somewhat ironic that, as philosophers and other intellectuals became more marginalized in general, those prepared to play a role in managing the most concrete decisions about life and death were often welcomed.

How, then, might philosophy be changed by the role of some of its scholars in the healthcare system? One important effect occurred in the 1970s when, in Stephen Toulmin's felicitous phrase, "medicine saved the life of ethics" (1986). Toulmin was referring to the rush of excitement about normative ethics which followed the discovery that there is genuine philosophical material in modern medicine. Thus was philosophical ethics saved from the doldrums after decades of "analytic" or "meta-ethics," an approach that concentrated only on the meaning of the terminology of morality, like "right" and "good."

Apart from the reemergence of normative ethics, the subject matter of moral philosophy itself shows signs of historic change inspired by the intercourse of philosophy and disease. The noted philosopher Baruch Brody has begun to develop a pluralistic approach to clinical ethical decision making he calls the "method of moral appeals" (Brody, 1988). A still more fundamental shift is represented in the work of another philosopher experienced in the hospital setting, Martin Benjamin, who has written extensively on the ethics of compromise (1990). Also in this period I, along with several others, became interested in the moral status of consensus in clinical decision making.

A common feature of these recent preoccupations among philosophers interested in bioethics is the way in which theory has begun to emerge from the mundane hospital experience. This is a reversal of the situation of bioethics in the 1970s and early 1980s, when philosophical theories were "applied" to clinical dilemmas. Not only in bioethics but in academic philosophy generally, there has been a modest rebellion against "methodism," the notion that if one can merely discover the correct philosophical method a conclusion will deductively emerge. Part of the criticism, articulated especially by Richard Rorty (1979), is the view that traditional moral philosophy was preoccupied with a Platonic notion of the good that is hopelessly divorced from the everyday understanding of better or worse instrumentalities. Alasdair MacIntyre's claim that moral frameworks must be located in particular cultural experiences is another aspect of this critique (MacIntyre, 1981).

Thus, just as major philosophical theorists in the 1980s were advocating a drastically more contextual approach to moral theorizing, their colleagues were being invited to assist the health care team with their deliberations in the clinical setting. The decade just past has therefore been one in which a confluence of conditions has enabled both the liberation of the conceptual material implicit in clinical ethics and the possibility that this experience will have a far greater influence on philosophy generally than even the renaissance of normative ethics in the 1970s.

WHO TEACHES VIRTUE?

In return for the privilege of attendance at the bedside, what does the philosopher have to offer? This is a raging controversy in bioethics, though in my experience it is one that lives more in conversation among clinically engaged philosophers than in print. The standard thinking about this question can be captured in two further questions: Can (medical) virtue be taught? And is the philosopher the one to do the teaching, or if not the philosopher, who should?

It happens that these questions have vexed philosophers since Socrates. I believe that they are in fact an unproductive way to characterize the nature of clinical ethics teaching. Thus, one critique of bioethics in the 1980s noted that, since moral virtue is supposed to be learned at one's parents' knees, any further instruction that one requires in this regard by the time of adulthood must be regarded as remedial at best. Moreover, it is not at all clear who can manage this remediation: since even parents often fail at moral education, in spite of their far greater opportunity to pursue it with their children, why should it be thought that a few hours of lectures from a professional philosopher will quicken a medical student's conscience?

The traditional reaction to this quandary in medical education is that of the "role model." The rationale is that, since instruction in morality for adults will fail if it is presented in a highly cognitive manner, it is best to expose the student to a model of probity in physician behavior. Ideally this is a senior doctor whose years of experience with human suffering have fostered equanimity and wisdom. This technique, part of the socialization process of young doctors for centuries, probably worked fairly well for a long time. Problems set in when the role models themselves came to have doubts about their ability to evaluate the complex set of options that modern medical technology offers them and their patients, options undreamt of by their distinguished predecessors. Ironically, but admirably, many of these reflective physicians began to model their own perplexity to their students. Some of them became energetic advocates of the study of ethics in the clinical setting. What, then, did they come to advocate? And what is it about the trained philosopher that qualifies him or her to provide this service? There are numerous multifaceted accounts of the goals of clinical ethics and the role of the philosopher. I will here offer my own construction, which I believe to be largely compatible with most of these accounts.

There are many aspects of medical practice for which the four years of medical school and several years of residency normally do not provide sufficient preparation. Put simply, the technical education of the physician-in-training barely hints at the swirl of social controversy around the practice of medicine. At the very least, medical students should be made aware of these controversies in a systematic manner. For example, students are impressed with the imperative to intervene with the best that medicine has to offer but are often shocked to discover that patients are often resistant, or even hostile, to their ministrations. They should be prepared for the encounter with patients or families that are not passive recipients of medical attention. One way to prepare them for this experience is to explain the changing historical conditions of doctor-patient relations in jurisprudential, financial, and sociological terms.

More specifically, the imperative to intervene has been given its unique modern impetus by the remarkable expansion of the medical armamentarium. But this has taken place during a period in which individual self-determination has also asserted itself in an equally unprecedented manner, the most obvious expression of this trend being the various civil rights movements. Physicians who practice in this society will inevitably have to come to grips with this paradox. The doctrine of informed consent can be presented as an attempt to reconcile these tensions and not merely as a hedge against liability.

Now what uniquely qualifies philosophers to take on this educational job? The answer, I believe, is that nothing *uniquely* qualifies the philosopher. Anyone comfortable with the free play of ideas, capable of formulating and assessing arguments, sensitive to connections between seemingly unrelated subjects, and with sufficient intellectual curiosity and self-confidence to become engaged with a variety of technical languages, can take this on. It does happen that, among the academic disciplines, philosophers are likely to have been trained specifically in the acquisition of these skills and to be self-selected in the possession of the necessary qualities (Moreno, 1991). Clearly, however, individuals from a variety of backgrounds, including law, medicine, or nursing, could be equally qualified.

I find that it is in the clinical setting—as compared to the lecture hall—that my lack of formal training in health science is both my greatest disadvantage and, curiously, my greatest advantage. The disadvantages are plain: clinicians may be skeptical that I can appreciate the burden of responsibility for the care of a human being who is ill, and my lack of systematic medical education often requires that I ask numerous clarifying questions about technical matters. These liabilities are not so severe as they might at first seem, however. Knowing that not all physicians who specialize in medical ethics are still in active practice or ever have been, clinicians liable to view me with skepticism sometimes view these physician-ethicists in the same way. Furthermore, I have found that physician-ethicists with medical backgrounds other than that pertinent to the case at hand (e.g., the internist consulting on a neonatal case) are often nearly as ignorant about technical details as I am. This is testimony to the fact that, as others have observed, medicine is no longer one profession, but many.

There are, moreover, some considerable advantages to my "uninitiated" status. First, there are no grounds for professional jealousy between a philosopher and a physician in the exercise of his or her normal duties. As a distinguished lay colleague once said to me, "The physicians don't worry that I'll take their case away." Second, sometimes in my relative ignorance of the medical details, I will ask a question too embarrassingly elementary for the younger physicians to ask but upon which the treatment decisions turn. More than once after raising such a question I have witnessed what was supposed to be an ethics conference turn into a medical education session for the benefit of the residents or even a debate among senior clinicians about the implications of previous cases or underlying theory. Third, there seems to be a useful role for a layperson who is acquainted with the clinical setting and conversant with its realities to articulate the patient's point of view to physicians who feel terribly frustrated by the environment of contemporary practice. To borrow from an infamous and frustrated query of Sigmund Freud, a question on the minds of many physicians these days is "What do patients want?" Finally, there are specific advantages for the philosopher as compared to the lawyer in this role, for lawyers are commonly so stereotyped by physicians that it can be difficult for them to be heard as sympathetic or at least neutral. Philosophers can occupy a certain moral high ground, the same high ground that theologians used to be able to claim before our hopelessly pluralistic value system began to undermine their claim to voice a moral consensus.

All this is not to deny that my lay status sometimes subjects me to dismissal out-of-hand by physicians. Following a grand rounds presentation in which I suggested that physicians who adopt paternalistic attitudes toward their patients would not tolerate those same attitudes if they were directed at them by an attorney they had retained, a physician rose to suggest that neither would an airline pilot accept advice from a passenger in a mid-air emergency. I replied that the pertinent question is not how the plane is flown but where it shall go. Regardless of the cogency of my reply, however, I am fairly sure that physician-ethicists are less liable to find themselves the subject of such a lecture. An anecdote told to me by a philosopher colleague makes the point more simply and directly: "I don't know anything about ethics," a senior physician said after a subtle philosophical analysis of a moral dilemma, "I just try to help people."

For all the uncertainty about the nature of clinical ethics in general and the role of the hospital philosopher in particular, there is no doubt that the coming years will see even more interest in this work. The State of Maryland has long required all its hospitals to have an ethics committee. Every major certifying specialty board includes questions on ethics in its examination, and in most specialties medical ethics education is required of accredited programs. Every year more major academic medical centers create new appointments in clinical ethics, and curricular offerings in medical ethics and medical humanities continue to proliferate.

Clinical ethics is a professional pursuit that has grown in demand without a clear prior understanding of precisely what qualifies one to provide this service. For some time there has been an assumption that the philosopher, at least, was qualified by virtue of his or her understanding of the great moral theories. But I have detected decreasing satisfaction with the notion that in practice the great philosophies can simply be applied to real cases of human suffering, a level of concreteness for which they were not designed. I have found that the knowledge of ethical theory is only one of a number of elements that help me to work with healthcare providers. Another aspect of my philosophical education that is most helpful is the ability to analyze a conceptual problem in a way that may clarify the issues. By contrast, while there are those who argue that the clinical ethicist's role should be that of Socratic "facilitator of moral inquiry," simply asking difficult questions without providing some guidance only aggravates an already frustrating situation.

But work on ethical problems directly with health care professionals in the real setting of healthcare delivery requires a further range of skills that have little to do with traditional training in any single discipline, including philosophy. One must be acquainted with relevant statutory and case law, the institutional structure of the healthcare system, the financing of health care, and the prevailing consensus and current issues in health policy. Some understanding of the economics of health care is very useful, and an appreciation for the sociological and political processes of the clinical setting is essential. Finally, sound interpersonal skills, particularly tactfulness and the ability to mediate among deeply felt differences while honoring them, can vastly enhance the value of the ethics consultant.

This list of skills suggests that it is no part of the job to reform any personal moral inadequacies that professionals might have. My understanding of what I do is pragmatic, and my estimate of its affects is modest: the teaching of ethics in the professional setting is not remedial moral education. Rather than personality change, a successful "ethics intervention" can work at a strictly cognitive level, providing information, articulating alternative courses of action, and offering standards for evaluation. Behavior change of some sort usually follows, even if it only has to do with a better understanding of the legal system; and if changed moral attitudes or greater personal virtue ensues, that is more of a matter of luck than wisdom.

Thus, I cling to a healthy philosophical doubt about what I do even as the demand increases, even as I know that hardly anyone is "trained" for this job of ethics consultation. As has so often been noted, our values are playing "catch-up" with the promises, uncertainties, and costs of the modern medical armamentarium. Yet to say this is perhaps to let us all off the hook too easily. That is, my greatest worry is that I am part of an elegant, functional distraction from the underlying shortcomings of the healthcare system. For at least many of the problems that present themselves as ethical in the acute hospital situation are artifacts of structural arrangements that derive from political processes.

For example, the low-birth-weight infants that crowd our intensive care nurseries are instances of preventable suffering. By focusing on a range of tragic choices after the fact, we miss the background of poor prenatal care that is partly a function of politically driven allocation arrangements. The same can be said about ethical dilemmas in the distribution of donor or artificial organs: wouldn't it be better to attend to public health strategies that discourage self-destructive behaviors like smoking and drinking? Or consider the heated debates about terminating high-tech life-sustaining treatment: wouldn't they be less pressing if there were no financial imperative to deliver virtually every gravely ill person to a hospital, where, often regardless of their expressed wishes, they will likely be intubated and sustained indefinitely?

In this country we manage to turn each decision into an isolated dilemma or to turn every uncertainty into a zero-sum ethics game in which there is a right or a wrong. While I relish the extraordinary opportunity I have been given as a member of this generation of philosophers, I struggle with the limitations of particularity in a way that never hampered the great universal metaphysicians, at least not in their treatises. Consolation I find in James, the physician who never practiced, the philosopher with a medical degree, the quintessential American:

> Hands off: neither the whole of truth nor the whole of good is revealed to any single observer, although each observer gains a partial superiority of insight from the peculiar position in which he stands. Even prisons and sick rooms have their special revelations. It is enough to ask of each of us that he should be faithful to his own opportunities and make the most of his own blessings, without presuming to regulate the rest of the vast field. (1968, 645)

3

Arguing Euthanasia

In 1974, several months before my twenty-second birthday, my mother and I were forced to make some agonizing decisions. My father, then in his mid-eighties, collapsed following a severe case of the flu. During the next few weeks he became more and more disoriented, the result of a series of tiny strokes that he had suffered over a period of time but whose cumulative effects were gradually overcoming his recuperative powers. Finally, he stopped eating and drank only enough to keep his mouth moist.

My father was a physician, and he and my mother had made a pact that, should he become seriously ill, she would not send him to the hospital to die. His wishes stemmed from fifty years of professional experience with large institutions and from his distress at the hospital death of his mother some years before. Fortunately, we were in a position to honor his preference. Early in his illness we installed a hospital bed in his room so that he would not fall while sleeping. Nursing care was available around the clock.

As my father's condition worsened, however, his discomfort grew. Barely coherent, he seemed to reverse his earlier wishes and began asking to be taken to the hospital. At that point his private physician, an old friend and colleague, determined that he was terminally ill and suggested that he be given regular morphine injections. When his doctor asked him if he wanted morphine he shook his head, but he continued to complain of discomfort. The next day, we urged his doctor to give him the injection without asking. Though conscious, this time my father acquiesced to what would be the first of many such injections. Finally, he became composed and comfortable, and a few weeks later he passed away quietly.

Our own uncertainty had added to the trauma of the situation. When his pain became intense and he asked to go to the hospital, we had to decide whether this was an authentic request or rather a cry for help. Believing that she knew his true wishes, my mother tried first to relieve his pain. But his initial reluctance to be medicated raised other questions: Did he fear the further clouding of his intellect? Or, in his deluded state, did he think he was being given an overdose? Or did he perhaps simply fail to recognize his old colleague? The decision to proceed with the injection the next day was also fraught with danger: What if he physically resisted? Would we have him restrained and injected against his apparent will on the grounds that he was confused and deluded? We were trying to help him, but would a second attempt at injection make him less trusting of us in his final days?

Although the story of my father's death seems straightforward in retrospect, at several points it could have gone very differently. If my father had been admitted to the hospital, if his doctor had expressed reluctance about pain medication, or if we had not suggested a more aggressive approach to the injection, his course would have drastically changed. Today, for medical, practical, and legal reasons, it is less likely that a physician would be willing to take care of such a patient outside the hospital. But my father knew that his chances of dying peacefully would have been lessened in the hospital. Though technical interventions were limited then as compared to twenty years later, my father did not want to spend his last days in an impersonal institutional environment. Today routine end-of-life hospital care tends to be even more aggressive then it was then. In fact, after his suffering was under control, my father gave no indication that he wanted to leave our home or that he wanted the medication to cease. In the time that followed, a legion of old friends and former students were able to visit and say good-bye, unimpeded by hospital technology or visiting hours.

That my father's dying unfolded as it did was due to several factors: his communication of his wishes to my mother, the availability of medical and nursing care at home, the financial wherewithal to afford such services, my mother's exceptional courage and determination, and an era when institutionalized and technologically mediated death could be more easily avoided. Even as recently as the mid-1970s, physicians were less inclined to practice defensive medicine for legal reasons, and end-of-life technology could not so effectively extend the dying process. Perhaps most important was that we knew my father well enough to assess his true wishes accurately when we needed to. I have often wondered how differently things would have gone if any one of these factors had been absent.

I have wondered, too, if we made the right decision in the first place about keeping him at home. Should we have hospitalized him in spite of his previously expressed wish? In doing so we might have had him for a few more months, though in an increasingly debilitated condition. Or, if he was ready to die, would he have preferred to have his trusted medical friend end it quickly with a lethal dose? Or, as a strong-willed man, would he have elected to give himself the injection when still able do it? As a licensed physician, he had access to the medication for an overdose, but because of his zest for life, I doubt if he ever considered death by his own hand. Perhaps he would have preferred his doctor to give him a lethal injection, as in the case of his medical school lecturer Sigmund Freud. Even under the best of circumstances, dying can be a grueling and laborious affair. At one point, after weeks spent lying in bed, he said to my mother, "It takes a long time to die."

Mainly I feel that we did well by my father, but doubt is a humane and noble thing when the stakes are so high.

As much as any other personal factor, the experience of my father's dying led me to a career as a teacher and scholar of medical ethics. The subject of euthanasia and assisted suicide is among the most ancient and important in this field. The Hippocratic Oath, which remains the primary touchstone of medical ethics in our culture, appears to rule out physician-assisted death. But it is reasonable to ask how a code that is over two thousand years old can apply to medical techniques that would have been beyond the wildest dreams of its author. In fact, for a few hundred years, and perhaps longer, some patients have called the strict Hippocratic prohibition into question, and it is certain that some doctors have violated it.

Of course, it is one thing to say that a moral code like the Hippocratic Oath is often violated and quite another thing to say that it is wrong. But the fact is that the oath is among the most revered and least read documents of Western civilization, even among physicians. Many medical school commencements include a ritualistic recitation of the oath by the young men and women about to become doctors of medicine, but it is usually a sanitized version that omits references to sensitive subjects like euthanasia and abortion. Ignorance of the Hippocratic Oath's actual content is perhaps best exemplified by the frequent references to the maxim *Primum non nocere,* or "First do no harm." The precept is indeed Hippocratic, but it does not appear in the oath.

One could argue that our modern technology and our complex society have left the oath's ancient wisdom far behind, that what worked twenty-three hundred years ago cannot work now. But even then the Hippocratic circle was but one of many medical cults; and dissatisfaction with its apparent prohibition of physician-assisted suicide, or active euthanasia, is nothing new. In his *Utopia* (1516), Thomas More wrote:

> They console the incurably ill by sitting and talking with them and by alleviating whatever pain they can. Should life become unbearable for the incurables the magistrates and priests do not hesitate to prescribe euthanasia. . . . When the sick have been persuaded of this, they end their lives willingly either by starvation or drugs, that dissolve their lives without any sensation of death. Still, the Utopians do not do away with anyone without his permission, nor lessen any of their duties to him.

Of course, the social conditions under which most people get sick and die are still far short of utopia, which gives rise to legitimate concerns about the implications of such a practice in the real world.

It is interesting that the modern secular state has mainly avoided the issue. Euthanasia and assisted suicide have usually been treated as forms of homicide, at least technically, and only in the Netherlands have the courts officially tolerated the practice. But all that changed dramatically on November 8, 1994, when Oregon voters became the first in the nation to approve a ballot measure that allows doctors to hasten the death of those who are terminally ill. Measure 16 was the successor to two narrowly defeated initiatives in Washington State in 1991 and in California (for the second time) in 1992. Importantly, those previous efforts permitted a doctor to administer lethal drugs, while the Oregon law only allows a physician to prescribe an overdose of medication. If Measure 16 survives a constitutional challenge in court, it will legalize physician-assisted suicide in Oregon, not active euthanasia, and this is thought to be less liable to abuse. In the Netherlands, allegations that some patients have been put to death without their consent are the basis for powerful criticisms of the Dutch courts' toleration of active euthanasia.

With the approval of the Oregon initiative, an epochal legal, cultural, and psychological barrier has been breached for better or for worse. Evaluation of the actual results of the law will surely take years, but it may take far less time for other states to approve similar measures now that the line has been crossed. It is therefore critical to understand how we arrived at this Northwest passage.

The popular movement that led up to the Oregon referendum can be dated from at least 1988, when the *Journal of the American Medical Association* published an anonymous 500-word article called "It's Over, Debbie." The author claimed to be a physician in a graduate training program who had granted the apparent wish of a seemingly dying young woman to be put out of her misery.

The brief entry unleashed a firestorm of criticism from some of the country's leading medical ethicists, perhaps especially those who were physicians. Their outrage was directed primarily at the reported conduct of the doctor. According to the article, he or she had met this patient only minutes before the event, and in the middle of the night, without even a modicum of standard assessment and consultation. In the critics' judgment, the act described was without the slightest shred of professionalism—a thoughtless murder perpetrated against a vulnerable person in a hospital bed, in wholesale violation of the most elementary standards of medical ethics. The ethicists unleashed a secondary volley at the editor of the prestigious journal for even having published such a document.

A backlash ensued among professionals and members of the general public who were unimpressed by the alleged wisdom of these ethicists; they upbraided the ethics experts for failing to take adequate account of the suffering of the dying. During the 1980s, many people had become sensitized to the contemporary problems of dying. Indeed, stories about dying people had almost become a literary genre. Among them was journalist Betty Rollin's powerful description, in her book *Last Wish* (1998), of her mother's struggle with terminal cancer and of her decision to assist in her mother's suicide. There were also well-publicized double suicides by aging couples, including that of cultural critic Arthur Koestler, author of *Darkness at Noon* (1984), and his wife.

If the ethicists felt themselves to be taking a principled, even if not wholly popular, stand in the "Debbie" case, there were soon further frontal assaults on the conventional wisdom. Timothy Quill, a respected Rochester, New York, physician, reported in the *New England Journal of Medicine* (1991) that he had prescribed barbiturates to a woman suffering from cancer, knowing that she intended to use them to commit suicide. There was nothing anonymous about this report, and unlike the Debbie case, which struck some as a hoax designed to spur discussion, Quill's story about "Diane" had the ring of truth. Most challenging to the prevailing wisdom was the fact that Quill had a long-term professional relationship with Diane and that she had been found free of clinical depression, both thought to be key factors in any justifiable physician-assisted suicide (typically accomplished by the patient's using prescription medication authorized by the cooperating doctor). In contrast, Debbie was the subject of active euthanasia—accomplished in a deliberate and lethal act by the physician. Debbie was not only actively killed, but many psychiatrists pointed out that she might have been clinically depressed and therefore unable to rationally assess her situation. On the whole, Quill's approach struck many physicians as the least objectionable form of physician-assisted death; this rendered it a respectable option for some patients.

The growing public debate was further inflamed and complicated by the controversial publication of *Final Exit* (2002) by Derek Humphry. Humphry is the founder of the Hemlock Society, an organization that advocates making the option of suicide available to all who suffer and wish to end their lives. A how-to suicide manual, *Final Exit* quickly became a best-seller that put the basics of relatively efficient self-destruction into the hands of nonphysicians.

Then, as if on cue, a retired pathologist named Jack Kevorkian designed a Rube Goldberg–style "suicide machine" that he made available to numbers of persons who were suffering from progressive terminal diseases such as Alzheimer's. The fact that Kevorkian held a medical degree somewhat obscured the fact that his technique was more a matter of engineering than of clinical sophistication. But each of Kevorkian's assisted deaths grabbed headlines. His court battles and jail time transformed him into an odd sort of folk hero who symbolized a populist protest against the medical-legal bureaucracy that seems to stand between the individual and his or her freedom of choice. To many, Kevorkian's was the ultimate act of fighting city hall.

Ironically, the capstone of an evolving moral consensus on end-of-life treatment, the U.S. Supreme Court's decision in the case of Nancy Cruzan (1990), occurred just as this highly publicized and hotly controversial series of incidents was getting under way. Cruzan was a young Missouri woman who had sustained a traumatic head injury in an automobile accident. She survived for years in a "persistent vegetative state" (PVS), the same condition into which Karen Quinlan had lapsed. Patients who are PVS have lost the neurophysiological basis for consciousness. They have sleep-wake cycles and open their eyes, and sometimes they moan, but they have no awareness of their surroundings or of themselves. Their reactions to the world are based entirely on reflex.

Unlike the Quinlans, who asked only for the removal of the artificial breathing apparatus, Nancy Cruzan's parents wanted to withdraw the feeding tubes that were keeping their daughter alive. The Cruzans believed that their daughter would not have wanted to be kept alive in this way; they appealed to the Missouri courts to permit them to satisfy what they believed would have been Nancy Cruzan's wish, to be permitted to die. But the state's supreme court ruled that the available evidence was not clear and convincing about Nancy Cruzan's preferences—the standard of evidence required in Missouri in such a case. The Cruzans decided to appeal the decision to the U.S. Supreme Court, which delivered its ruling in 1990.

In *Cruzan* the Supreme Court upheld a state's right to require a high standard of evidence about an incompetent patient's previous wishes concerning life-sustaining treatment. Though that decision was regarded as a setback by some patients' rights advocates, the justices also articulated the well-recognized right of a competent patient to decline any and all treatment, including life-sustaining treatment. This was a first for the high court. Furthermore, from a legal point of view, the justices settled a question that had been a hot spot of medical ethics debate in the 1980s—whether artificial feeding counted as a form of medical therapy that (like a ventilator) could be declined in advance. The court concluded that feeding tubes are a high-tech treatment that may not be forced on a patient, even though the obvious outcome will be starvation.

The Cruzans lost the battle but won the war. Back home, a court-appointed guardian for Nancy determined that new information about her wishes was indeed clear and convincing. The feeding tubes were removed, and Nancy Cruzan died. The critical point in the aftermath of *Cruzan* is this: *the legal right to decline life-sustaining treatment after one is no longer conscious clearly applies to artificial feeding.* This landmark decision appears to certify that, in the United States, patients may decline any and all life-sustaining treatment, even if they become unconscious—a legal right that can be accepted even by those who reject active euthanasia or physician-assisted suicide.

To many in the medical ethics community, the undisciplined public debate about euthanasia that arose around the time of the court's decision threatened to disrupt the carefully wrought consensus, culminating in *Cruzan,* about patients' rights to forgo life-sustaining treatment. Though these rights had long been recognized in the common law for competent patients, clinical realities often involve patients like Nancy Cruzan who have lost the capacity to decide. Progress toward the emerging doctrine that *formerly competent* patients did not lose this right had effectively begun with the *Quinlan* decision in 1976, which assured the right of a permanently unconscious patient to forgo artificial breathing. A presidential commission on ethical problems in medicine strongly concurred in 1982, and this is the view that crystallized decisively in *Cruzan.*

But now, after all this work to assure the rights of patients who are no longer competent to forgo end-of-life treatment, some worried that the clamor for more active control over dying would both obscure and jeopardize the real progress that had been made. In fact, the state of Michigan enacted a statute, aimed at Kevorkian, that many thought went too far by inhibiting appropriate patient decisions to forgo treatment.

Strictly speaking, the term *euthanasia* refers to actions or omissions that result in the death of a person who is already gravely ill. Techniques of active euthanasia range from gunfire to lethal injection, while passive euthanasia can be achieved by failing to treat pneumonia or by withholding or withdrawing ventilatory support. The current medical ethics consensus has thus implicitly legitimized *voluntary* passive euthanasia. This consensus relies on the moral legitimacy of letting the underlying disease process take its natural course, if that is what the patient would have wanted. Although many do not find passive euthanasia to satisfy the idea of a "good death" (eu-thanasia), most prefer it to lengthening the dying process due to human intervention.

Yet this consensus is fairly narrow, and at its margins there are problems. Although passive euthanasia against the patient's wishes (*involuntary* euthanasia) is clearly prohibited by the current consensus, passive euthanasia in the absence of knowledge of the patient's wishes (*nonvoluntary* euthanasia) remains controversial. Moreover, some acts of euthanasia are hard to classify. Some of those who can accept withdrawal of ventilatory support if wanted by the patient (a clear case of passive voluntary euthanasia) nevertheless reject the withdrawal of feeding tubes, even at the patient's request. In spite of the Supreme Court's decision in *Cruzan,* this difference of opinion is not likely to disappear.

Within the meaning of *active* euthanasia, the difference between *voluntary* euthanasia and *nonvoluntary* euthanasia is also important. Active voluntary euthanasia is performed at the patient's request, while active nonvoluntary euthanasia may be performed on a patient who is not competent and who has not requested it. There is also active *involuntary* euthanasia, which refers to "mercy killing" done against the patient's wishes. Although hardly anyone advocates active involuntary euthanasia, some worry that we are on the "slippery slope" to such exterminations, perhaps on a Nazi-like, eugenic basis. In any case, when advocates talk about euthanasia, they can generally be assumed to mean the kind that is voluntary, with the passive variety far less controversial than the active. And all those who advocate that dying patients should be permitted to die when they wish endorse assisted suicide.

In spite of the ethicists' conviction that the humane abatement of life-sustaining treatment can and should be kept distinct from the active-euthanasia and assisted-suicide debate, their critics assert that the drift toward more deliberate means of ending life is a natural consequence of the slippery slope represented in the triumph of autonomy. In reply, it should be pointed out that our society has in fact clambered *up* the slope, toward greater scrutiny of end-of-life treatment than was true a generation ago, when most Americans died under the supervision of doctors who were left largely to their own devices. In those days, passive euthanasia, with or without knowledge of the patient's wishes, was probably far more common than it is today. Many senior physicians recall cases of dying elderly patients who could not feed themselves but were comfortable. It was regarded as inhumane to force-feed them and extend their dying process. Instead, a glass of water was placed next to their night table with the rationale, "If she wants to take a drink, she will."

Yet slippery slopes cannot easily be dismissed in an era when the boundaries of life are being technologically challenged at both ends. Human life with test tube origins is now a commonplace. We will shortly be in a position not only to avoid giving birth to children with certain terrible afflictions but also to design individuals with genetically engineered desirable characteristics. Try as we might to set limits on future manipulations of chromosomes, the genies of applied science are notoriously difficult to put back into their lamps, as the atomic age attests. One simply cannot predict whether, or how, a society with so much control over the beginning of life will seek to control its end.

Clearly, the recent euthanasia debate has incorporated a wider subject area than euthanasia per se. Assisted suicide, and especially physician-assisted suicide, has come within the ambit of the controversy, even though it does not fall within the strict meaning of *euthanasia,* and even though the term *suicide* has pejorative implications that *euthanasia* does not have. Although one might object to this development on semantic grounds, it does reflect the fact that modern medical interventions have themselves obscured the difference between euthanasia and suicide. Take the example of a competent patient with end-stage emphysema. If she insists on the cessation of ventilatory support, is that euthanasia or suicide? Moreover, if a decision is made to medicate the patient so that she does not experience suffocation, is that appropriate therapy or physician-assisted suicide?

Advances in life-sustaining technology include ventilators, artificial feeding, and advanced cardiac life support. There have also been vast improvements in life-*extending* technologies, such as cancer chemotherapy and, allegedly, the drug AZT for AIDS. Although the life-extending therapies are not usually directly implicated in euthanasia debates, they have created a novel sort of dependence on the medical system previously unknown to patients who were, in some sense, dying. Thus, some have asserted that a physician has an obligation to do more than cease providing such treatment when the patient wishes it to stop; after all, the patient's life has been extended by this intervention, and so has his suffering. Shouldn't the physician then advance the moment of death at the patient's request? And if she refuses, isn't this a form of abandonment?

In part, this aspect of the debate has turned on a disagreement about the ways in which dying patients actually suffer and the extent to which that suffering can be alleviated. Those who object to the termination of food and fluids argue that no one should undergo starvation, while experts in hospice care contend that, properly managed, this is among the least uncomfortable ways to die. Those who object to abandoning a terminal cancer patient to the disease's natural end state note the pain she will endure, while experts in palliative care claim that proper pain management can be applied to all but the most intractable cases without resort to active euthanasia.

The moral significance of a dying person's pain has also been subject to philosophical disagreement. The philosopher James Rachels famously argued that active euthanasia may actually be morally preferable to passive euthanasia if the patient will suffer during a drawn-out process of natural death (1986). Others have wondered how broadly the idea of pain should be construed: Does the knowledge that one is facing a gradually degenerative course, as in the case of amyotrophic lateral sclerosis (Lou Gehrig's disease), create so much mental suffering that this is a rational reason to consider suicide? What about the person suffering from years of chronic depression that has proven refractory to treatment?

The question of whether a suicide can ever be rational falls into the boundary of psychiatry and philosophy. In general, the two literatures agree that, while suicide hardly ever meets the criteria of rationality, it cannot be ruled out in all cases. Philosophically, a rational assessment of one's prospects might, in theory, yield the calculation that an end to one's life is more valuable (for oneself and for those one loves) than continuing life with burdens that cannot be compensated by other experiences. Psychiatrically, although depression typically accompanies suicidal ideation, it cannot be said always to accompany such thoughts. In any case, even if the suicidal act does not meet the highest standards of rationality, the contention that one has a moral *right* to suicide is different: Whose life is it anyway?

In the largest sense, the euthanasia debate has been energized in the modern world by the insistence in recent medical ethics on patient self-determination. The abortion debate, too, reflects the influence of the self-determination principle. Abortion may also share with euthanasia the distinction of being one of the most ancient medical ethics issues, given the explicit mention of both in most versions of the Hippocratic Oath. The euthanasia debate differs from the conflict over abortion in crucial ways, however. It has not been so extremely, and perhaps hopelessly, politicized as abortion, and it does not involve allegations of a second, innocent life. Rather, euthanasia, and especially physician-assisted suicide, appears as the ultimate postmodern demand for personal dignity in an era of technologically mediated death.

If I could commend one critical question to the reader, it would be this: Given both the inevitability of death and the fact that human arrangements rarely satisfy human aspirations, can a system of physician-assisted dying satisfy individual preferences without degrading values that are abstract but of continuing importance? Put differently: Are there circumstances under which assisted suicide or euthanasia would leave unharmed, if not promote, life-oriented values?

Nietzsche thought so. In *Zarathustra*, the grandfather of postmodernism had his prophet declare his determination not to be like the "rope makers," who "drag out their threads behind them." Zarathustra called for a "free death," the only one that can "hallow the oaths of the living."

But there is another side of the Nietzschean tradition besides that of personal transcendence. Whether justly or not, for modern readers references to Nietzsche are often reminders of holocausts against defenseless innocents, and none is more vulnerable than the dying person. That vulnerability works both ways, of course: vulnerable to suffering as well as to harm. Some acts intended to prevent suffering may inadvertently cause still greater harm. Does euthanasia fall into that category? Or assisted suicide? I cannot think of a greater challenge to our wisdom or our humanity.

PART TWO

NATURALIZING BIOETHICS IN THEORY AND PRACTICE

Introduction

In my general introduction I alluded to my affection for the American philosophical tradition. Only a few "Americanists" in philosophy have found their way to bioethics. Most bioethicists cut their philosophical teeth on analytic or Continental philosophy, the dominant traditions in the academy. Those of us who identify with the kind of thinking represented in figures like Charles Peirce, William James, and John Dewey have had a hard time explaining why we find the contribution of the so-called pragmatists to be so appropriate for bioethics. The first chapter in this part is an attempt to provide that explanation, though as I indicate, I prefer the aspect of pragmatism known as naturalism when formulating my approach to bioethics.

Though this is far too simply put, *pragmatism* is a way of distinguishing between ideas or terms or theories, while *naturalism* is a worldview that a number of pragmatists have shared. So for the pragmatist, the difference between one theory and another turns on the predictions that each theory generates; if they don't differ in this respect, they are not meaningfully different. Pragmatism was deployed to attack the gobbledygook that too often passes for philosophy, but also to advance a connection between mentality and the realm of action. In other words, ideas are not separate from the world; they are active agents for use in the world.

The activist spirit implicit in the idea of pragmatism appealed to me, and the bioethicist is nothing if not an activist philosopher, whether in the clinic, the committee room, the advisory panel, or the op-ed pages. But over the years I have come to see naturalism as the still more profound philosophical point for bioethicists, the idea that human values are part of nature, not disconnected from it. That means that they arise from our experience and must be tested against experience. The bioethicist must take this attitude, it seems to me, especially in the context of policy. Yet while we must be willing to revise our ethical conclusions in light of experience, we must also hold firmly to them until they are clearly inadequate.

I have never seen the danger of relativism in this view, though it is the most ready stone to throw at naturalism. For the fact is that we do come to consciousness with certain very general moral values, and those who deviate from those general values (do not harm the innocent, try to promote the good, etc.) are unacceptable in any culture. Rather, what is far more difficult is knowing when and how to revise an ethical approach. That is the red meat of bioethics.

For the clinical ethicist, this problem comes up either as an individual consultant or as a member of a small group, an ethics committee. Each of these contexts is represented in the other two chapters in this section. They pose somewhat different problems for the clinical ethicist, problems that make the role a continuing puzzle and the subject of much talk among colleagues. No matter what our philosophical preferences are, puzzling and talking are things we do well.

4

Bioethics Is a Naturalism

I argue that bioethics is a naturalistic philosophy in the sense associated with the tradition of American philosophic naturalism and that the genealogy of bioethics as a predominantly American intellectual field helps account for bioethics as a naturalism. To offer these views is not to deny that there have been multiple intellectual influences on the origins of bioethics. It is patent that several faith traditions, especially Roman Catholicism, and several secular moral philosophic orientations, especially utilitarianism and deontology, have heavily influenced both the methods and the substance of modern biomedical ethics. It is also clear that bioethics has arisen in other national contexts, particularly in the United Kingdom and the Commonwealth countries, in western Europe, in some Latin American countries, and increasingly in central Europe.

Nevertheless, one of my premises in this chapter is that the social institution of bioethics has an undeniably American flavor and that bioethics is mainly an American field in its origins and, perhaps more controversially, in its style. By the latter claim I mean that bioethics emphasizes themes such as moral autonomy and pluralism and that in its practice, from calling for clinical ethics consultations to convening national ethics commissions, it is consensus oriented. In fact, a former director of the French equivalent to the U.S. National Institutes of Health has complained that bioethics commissions are so preoccupied with consensus that consensus is often forced on society (Moreno, 1996a). Although consensus is not exclusively American, American society is exceptional in being autonomy-driven in its ideology and pluralistic in its makeup. Perhaps for this reason, our public discourse is particularly preoccupied with the problem of achieving consensus (Moreno, 1995).[1]

Few bioethicists—and not all philosophers—have a firm grasp of the views associated with American philosophic naturalism. Therefore, I first need to explicate that philosophy, partly by distinguishing it from the somewhat more familiar epistemological naturalism associated with thinkers such as Willard van Orman Quine. I then move to an account of some ideas in ethical naturalism, after which I am in a position to explain more fully why I see bioethics as a naturalism.

AMERICAN PHILOSOPHIC NATURALISM

Although pragmatism may be regarded as a philosophic method, American philosophic naturalism is a worldview most closely identified with the writings of Charles S. Peirce, William James, John Dewey, George Herbert Mead, and Clarence Irving Lewis (Rosenthal, 1990). Both pragmatism and naturalism have come to be identified as well with the writings of a more recent distinguished philosopher, Willard van Orman Quine. However, the similarities and differences between what may be called *epistemological naturalism* and *philosophic naturalism* are instructive.

Both naturalisms reject *foundationalism,* the notion that knowledge must be grounded in a priori methods of inquiry. Versions of foundationalism are represented in many of the most influential philosophies, Platonism being the classic example. The natural-

---

1. In my book *Deciding Together: Bioethics and Moral Consensus* (1995), I elaborate a view of bioethics as a consensus-oriented enterprise.

isms find the same essential flaw in all philosophies that appeal to transcendent essences or structures: these philosophies fail to see that knowledge can—and in the final analysis must—be understood as embedded in the world of our experience rather than in some separate realm of being. Foundationalism is not only a failure to apprehend knowledge as "a natural phenomenon that must be examined in its natural setting" (Rosenthal, 1996); it is also a failure of nerve, a fruitless and even pathetic attempt to reach into some great and mysterious beyond for answers that can be attained only within experience.

Part of the appeal of foundationalism lies in its promise that the key to knowledge can be found without doing the hard work of inquiring into the world as it is. Rather, according to naturalist philosophers, there is no escaping the nitty-gritty of such work if any real knowledge is to be found. All else is a philosophical form of that emotional refuge known to psychologists as magical thinking. The classic critique of this poignant, ancient, but finally tragic quest for certainty is found in Dewey's critical work of that title (1929).

Both epistemological and philosophic naturalisms thus agree that a satisfactory account of the nature of knowledge can be achieved only by attending to the methods and techniques exemplified within experience, and that by so attending, an account can be given of the possibility of knowledge itself. In other words, the two great epistemological questions must be approached in a naturalistic spirit. The pragmatic element of this attitude should be apparent; indeed, it is a pragmatic temperament that leads one to a naturalistic worldview. Furthermore, when one engages in a naturalistic inquiry into knowledge by examining the ways in which it is actually attained, one notes certain means and patterns that are more productive in the pursuit of knowledge than others. These lessons are inherently normative in the sense that they provide guidance concerning the ways that the expansion of knowledge ought to be pursued. Some of these normative lessons have moral as well as instrumental implications insofar as they provide counsel about, for example, the most economic and therefore least wasteful ways to pursue what can be known.

Epistemological naturalism and American philosophic naturalism also agree that attention to the ways knowledge is gained shows a continuity between these means and the method of science itself. At this point, however, the two naturalisms begin to part company. The pragmatic temperament can be traced to a rejection of a "spectator" theory of knowledge associated with Cartesianism, the view that the observer stands apart from and over against the object of knowledge. The pragmatic naturalist understands that the knower and that which is known are in the same matrix, just as the inquirer is within nature and is one of its entities along with the object of knowledge, not outside of nature or fundamentally disconnected from the object.

Yet epistemological naturalism, for all its powerful contributions to modern philosophy, is too closely associated with causal theories of observation, such that causal processes are said to produce true belief-states. The psychological behaviorism of Quine, for example, is in the tradition of J. B. Watson and B. F. Skinner, who stressed a stimulus-response model that places observer and observed apart from each other in static relations. But the "behaviorism" of Mead and Dewey stresses the dynamic interaction of the knower with that which is to be known, the fact that the attitude (physical as well as psychological) of the inquirer influences the way the object is apprehended, just as the object influences the inquirer's experience. To use Dewey's phrase, the stimulus-response relation is not an arc, but a circuit (1971).

In rejecting epistemological naturalism, American philosophic naturalism also rejects the notion that the ultimate authority on the nature of the world is natural science and that the only questions that can legitimately be framed about the world must be expressed in the terms of natural science. The philosophic naturalist stresses the method of science rather than the content of science. Too great an emphasis on the content of science can lead to scientism, which is the substitution of dogma derived from current scientifically validated ideas for the open-minded inquiry and critical thinking characteristic of the method of science.

According to the philosophic naturalist, science can flourish only through an active engagement of the knower with the known, operating within the same matrix in a dynamic interaction through which emerge the meanings that make knowledge possible. More-over, the method of science does not result only in scientific infor-mation, and it is not used only in "scientific" contexts, for the method of science is mainly an intensified version of the patterns of successful investigation into any subject matter. Therefore, the meanings realized from inquiry may be the data typical of a sci-entific setting, but they may also be aesthetic signifiers or moral guides or some other type of information suitable to a certain type of inquiry.

Consistent with its conception of the dynamic interplay be-tween the knower and the known within the tissue of lived experi-ence, philosophic naturalism also emphasizes the experimental character of experience. Of course, not all experience is experi-mental in the systematic fashion of the method of science, but all experience is said to be continuous with that more intensified ver-sion characteristic of scientific inquiry. In fact, philosophic natur-alists contend that scientific investigation is rooted in the same tendencies that are brought to experience in general: stimulated by a problematic situation, the organism applies its various re-sources (prior experience, creative imagination, and so on) to the problem, implements a hypothetical solution, assesses the success of the endeavor, and, if necessary, formulates an alternative ap-proach.

Philosophic naturalism's rejection of the notion that only sci-ence can give a legitimate account of experience has been em-braced by another recent prominent philosopher whose views should not be too closely identified with naturalism. Richard Rorty rightly credits American naturalists, especially Dewey, for a pio-neering critique of foundationalism (1979). In elaborating his own version of that critique, Rorty has attracted more attention to some of Dewey's ideas than has been given to them for over fifty years. However, Rorty does not accept the philosophic natu-ralists' positive doctrine concerning the nature of experience and the intellectual tools inherent in experience. Hence Rorty con-tends, with the naturalists, that the content of science is only one way of representing the world, that it does not have sole license to confer legitimacy upon experience; but he does not appreciate that the method of science as intelligent inquiry has characteristics that inhere in all experience. Therefore, he is left to conclude that science is merely one sort of conversation among many, with none having any particular claim to priority.

Philosophic naturalists, while they agree that there is no privileged representation of experience, find within the method of science ways of knowing that are characteristic of all successful modes of representing experience, including the aesthetic and the moral. That is, not only scientific explorations but also artistic projects and ethical inquiries exhibit qualities of intelligent examination of the material provided by experience, including purposeful efforts at interpreting that material, revising it so that it bears the imprints of the examination, and engaging in further reconstructions in light of previous results. In other words, there are no hard-and-fast lines between different forms of inquiry into the nature of experience; each bears some characteristics of the others. In turn, these modes of inquiry into experience identify generic qualities of existence that extend well beyond the self-limited conditions established by the terms of even the most erudite conversation.

One element that the notion of conversation does capture is the social, and this is an important feature of philosophic naturalism, which views the interpersonal dimension as crucial for all modes of representing experience. Inquiry, whether scientific, aesthetic, or moral, is viewed as a social enterprise. The role of community is perhaps most apparent in science, wherein the opinion of a single investigator is subject to scrutiny by many colleagues who have the opportunity to confirm or disconfirm the hypothesis that has been proffered. Only when the community of inquirers reaches a consensus can the matter be said to have been settled, and even then it is settled only until no further doubt is raised.

In aesthetic affairs the success of a composition is dependent on the judgment of a community of appreciation, and in ethics the soundness of a principle or maxim of conduct depends on the judgment of a moral community. In a still more general sense, all forms of representation, all symbol systems and modes of signification, obviously require the cooperation of a linguistic community. In this respect the early American naturalists such as Peirce and James anticipated Ludwig Wittgenstein's famous private language argument, while Dewey, Mead, and Lewis elaborated its sociological and logical implications.

ETHICAL NATURALISM

The American philosophic naturalists wrote extensively about the implications of their views (which were by no means as uniform in their details as my very general summary might suggest) for many fields, including metaphysics, epistemology, logic, social and political philosophy, education, semiotics, and aesthetics. But it might well be that they had less to say about moral philosophy than about any other field. The most comprehensive anthology of writings central to American naturalism in the past fifty years, for example, includes only two selections on ethics, one of which was included in a volume published in 1944 (Krikorian), the other originally published in 1965 (Ryder, 1994).

One explanation for this relative lack of treatment of moral matters may be that American naturalists have been more interested in the process of inquiry, including inquiry into moral questions and the way society works out ethical quandaries, than in the big questions associated with classical moral philosophy, including what is the nature of the good? And what is the good life? Much of Dewey's theoretical ethics, for example, emerged through his writings on the nature of inquiry and community. Dewey's substantive ethical views appeared in his less technical essays—and in his social activism—related to concrete moral problems, such as his support of equality for women, his championing of civil liberties, and his opposition to American involvement in World War I.

Another reason for the paucity of commentary among American naturalists on ethical theory per se is that they do not accept the traditional agenda of moral philosophy, which engages in efforts to justify moral claims. The preferred form of justification is deductive, with one or more general moral principles comprising the major premise of an argument. But naturalists reject not only the a priori metaphysics of moral principles already noted but also the abstraction from actual moral experience represented in this conception of justification. Simply put, unless we are engaged in a mere academic exercise, we do not confront moral problems separate from our daily lives.

Actual moral problems are living problems and problems of living; they are "contexted" or embedded in states of affairs. Reminiscent of Aristotle's conception of practical wisdom, naturalists contend that actual moral problems call forth a wide range of skills, including a capacity to generalize from previous experience and an ability to project imaginatively what it would be like to select one alternative for action or the other. Context also helps determine our moral obligations, for what is an evident duty in one state of affairs is not at all apparent under another. Consider, for example, how the environment has been elevated to a moral concern in a short time by public awareness of such phenomena as the fragility of the ozone layer.

It is clear that American philosophic naturalists cannot accept the notion so important in so much modern ethical theory that there is a discrepancy between facts and values. The celebrated "naturalistic fallacy" is a fallacy only if expressed in a manner that begs the question, according to naturalists, for it is patent that in the world of experience moral judgment requires that one be informed of the facts. What kind of ethics is it that can afford to ignore actual states of affairs? One way to characterize the error inherent in the idea of the naturalistic fallacy is that it suggests there can be only one sort of relationship between facts and values—namely, a deductive one. The philosopher Owen Flanagan has noted that inductive and abductive processes are alternatives that the naturalist does well to select. Induction refers, of course, to generalization from previous experience, and abduction (a logic elaborated by Peirce) refers to the formulation of novel hypotheses based also on prior experience.

Even the idea that facts and values can be readily distinguished is doubtful, considering that facts are often, if not always, value laden and that values are often encountered as facts. The value-ladenness of assertions that are held up as fact is now a familiar phenomenon. Less familiar is the insight, associated especially with Dewey but also found in James's writings, that values are encountered in experience as features of states of affairs. The work of the cultural anthropologist is perhaps most consistently associated with values encountered in the field as facts in the worldview of a people. To turn those accounts upon ourselves (the inheritors of the western European worldview), the proposition that human rights are embedded in human dignity is so familiar as nearly to have lost its character as a value and claim authority as a fact.

Another prominent feature of ethical naturalism to which I have already alluded but which may be brought out more sharply is an emphasis on the situation or, perhaps a better term, the context of moral decision making. As has been said, what counts as a moral problem is tied up with a matrix of conditions that both define the problem and render it perceptible. For naturalists the context-dependent nature of moral choice is very nearly self-evident, for how else could any choice make contact with the issue at hand if it were not formulated in the light of the actual circumstances? Critics of naturalism may deride this approach as an invitation to "moral relativism," since it suggests that general principles or rules will have, at best, limited applicability in different situations. Naturalists embrace this conclusion. They especially see general rules or principles as providing orientation and guidance but also as carrying the seeds of dogmatism if not subject to interpretation in light of the facts of the case at hand. This position is entirely consistent with their view that inquiry requires openness, which is a methodological principle rather than a substantive general rule.

Similarly, naturalists regard choice as prior to rules in terms of actual experience. When faced with a concrete dilemma, moral or otherwise, people do not in fact consult theory, but they "apply themselves" to the problem. To be sure, this application of oneself includes application of what one knows about general rules, but it also includes application of one's experience with previous similar problems as well as judgment, intuition, temperament, and "gut feelings."

In other words, we bring to bear on an actual problem the greater or lesser part of the totality of our experience. An individual who literally consulted an ethics textbook when faced with a concrete dilemma would rightly be regarded as either naïve, obsessive, or simply lacking in understanding of the nature of ethical principles. Rather than implying a conclusion that must be drawn in particular cases, moral generalizations represent the retrospective aggregate of insights gleaned from eons of human experience—or so we hope. Whatever wisdom inheres in such generalizations cannot be deductively transferred to a problem at hand; rather, wisdom in the form of the judgment, or what Aristotle called practical wisdom, is also required in the assessment of the problematic situation with the aid of theory, rules, and principles.

By now it should be apparent why philosophic naturalists are not concerned with justification in the way that mainstream ethics has come to understand that as a part of its mandate. Principles do not justify a means of resolving a problem, moral or otherwise; only experience itself can do that. And in the real world any resolution always has a tentative quality, is always subject to revision. Only in a metaphysical fantasy are solutions permanent. The Good, therefore, is not a mere static thing, but a project— one that is undertaken, not by isolated individuals, but by social individuals, generally persons working together, even if often at odds. The Good, that which is desirable, is an ideal that helps organize human energies, which are in fact engaged in continuous social reconstruction. Conflict is frequently a feature of this process, but so is cooperation. Both conflict and cooperation are largely superficial qualities of social reconstruction, however. What is more important is the quality of the deliberation with which we have entered into the reconstructive process.

Like any dimension that calls on the method of inquiry, reconstruction requires intelligence, and in the world of actual human affairs it requires social intelligence. A socially intelligent response to a problematic situation that seems to require reconstruction resembles the method: understanding of the problem, a plan of action, a purpose or "end-in-view," and a willingness to engage in a further reconstruction if the hypothesized approach proves unsatisfactory.

These are among the crucial elements of ethical naturalism. It now remains to see not only how the field of bioethics exemplifies these elements but also how at least some of the practices associated with it might be viewed as a vindication of ethical naturalism.

BIOETHICS AS A NATURALISM

"By their fruits shall ye know them." This biblical admonition was cited by William James in one of his many attempts to define the pragmatic method. In this section I take a pragmatic view of the field of bioethics, for in ascertaining exactly what bioethics is, I am less concerned with how it is represented by its participants or commentators than with how it presents itself as an institution, a set of social practices.

The "practice" of bioethics occurs in numerous settings and groups: case conferences, ethics committees, classrooms, institutional review boards, print and broadcast media, professional organizations, bedside rounds, governmental panels, and civic organizations—and these do not exhaust the list. These settings and groups do have some elements in common, among the most important of which is that all of them involve communication, usually within a small group. This underscores the fact that bioethics is a social activity. Even when the ultimate goal is communication about an issue with a large group, such as members of a profession or the public in general, discussion tends to emanate from a relatively small number of initial participants.

It may be said that characterizing bioethics as a social activity is trivial, since by naturalism's own lights any intelligent activity is social. But the sociality I am referring to here is of the more quotidian variety. Compare the creative process in the traditional humanities disciplines with that of bioethics. It is a commonplace that humanistic creativity, while obviously profoundly influenced by teachers and contemporaries, has an ineluctably individual dimension. Put simply, it is the rare important document in the history of philosophy that has more than one author, and one that does is often labeled a manifesto. Yet important writings in bioethics appear regularly with multiple authors without prompting surprise.

One might argue that the difference can be explained by the relatively more fundamental concepts that are dealt with in philosophy, which require individual reflection, as compared to the concepts dealt with in an applied field such as bioethics. Apart from the fact that it is not always easy to tell which idea is more basic than another—and the problem of explaining why one sort of reflection calls upon individuality more than another—this account does not conflict with the observation that bioethical work, even in its written form, has a social character that the traditional humanities tend not to have.

As I have argued elsewhere (Moreno, 1995), the social character of bioethics is closely associated with its institutional functions. To see this, it is necessary to distinguish bioethics from the traditional humanistic disciplines in another way. Humanities professors may—and arguably should—leave their students in a state of doubt about some great human issues, such as the meaning of personhood or the significance of death. The Socratic tradition renders this view of humanistic pedagogy more than respectable.[2]

Bioethicists, too, may adopt the posture of the perpetual critic, but only insofar as they occupy the role of professor. To put it bluntly, those who leave the seminar room for the hospital conference room either drastically change their professional role or soon find themselves unwelcome or ineffective. Raising hard questions is important work, as is challenging prejudices and preconceptions and "speaking truth to power," but when action is required, as it is in virtually all the contexts in which medicine functions, the critical posture is simply not enough. Perhaps the most striking personal effect of bioethics on those who, like me, have undergone the transformation from humanities professor to bioethicist, is the way it forces those who might otherwise remain perpetual critics to "cash out" their views and take a position.

In framing matters in terms of their "cash value," I have made reference to the inherently pragmatic strain in bioethical practice. The naturalistic strain emerges insofar as the views that cash out are influenced as much by the problem at hand as by any prior theoretical views that participants bring to the table. In other words, it is rare (in my experience at least) to hear an ethics committee member explicitly appeal to the problem of balancing au-

---

2. For an expanded account of this way of viewing the tradition and an alternative view that is a near relation to the one I espouse, see Martha C. Nussbaum, *The Therapy of Desire* (1994).

tonomy and beneficence, for example. Rather, the facts of the case, its human importance, the medical uncertainty, the suffering involved, the legal and administrative complexities, and other more immediate factors tend to overwhelm theory.

To be sure, theory is often brought to bear on the problem at hand, but far more gingerly than is normally the case in the textbooks. And when theory is brought to bear, usually by oblique references or the shorthand use of terms such as self-determination, it bears none of the earmarks of deductive moral argument so dear to the hearts of many philosophical traditionalists. Instead there is a tentative and "hand-over-hand" quality to many of these conversations, with ethical theory one foothold among a precious few others, including prevailing practices, theological paradigms, institutional policies, useful analogies, and the law. Other resources are previous cases, and adumbrations suggested by casuistry in moral reasoning by Jonsen and Toulmin (1988), which has generated so much enthusiasm in the bioethical literature. These resources blend well with naturalism's emphasis on the moral guidance available in experience.

When ethical naturalists survey instances in which moral problems have been solved, they find that the most important resources are those that dwell within the situation rather than those that are introduced from outside of it. Principles are viewed, along with theories and other generalizations, as reducible to hypotheses about the realization of desirable outcomes. Among the resources inherent in the problematic situation are moral values themselves. When an ethical course is unclear, it is not owing to lack of moral options, but due to an excess of them. The challenge lies partly in ascertaining what outcome is both most desirable and within reach, then in constructing a means for its realization. Consider the example of physician-assisted suicide. What is wanted by all who dispute the matter is the most dignified death consistent with respect for life. Setting aside abstract recriminations about right and wrong, what concrete steps would be most likely to ensure the generally desired outcome?

I alluded to the casuistic explorations of Jonsen and Toulmin as compatible with a naturalistic bioethics. I now want to go further and argue that many of the arguments and accounts of bioethics are implicitly naturalistic, that the naturalistic orientation in bioethics is prevalent but unrecognized. A reliance on experience gleaned from previous cases is only one example, and one that has even been embraced by Tom Beauchamp and Jim Childress in the most recent edition of their influential text (2001). Other examples can be drawn from references to "species-typical functioning," as in debates about the meaning of health (Boorse, 1981), from attempts to rationally establish that fetuses have moral status through studies of fetal development (Knoppers and LeBris, 1991), from appeals to neuroanatomy in arguments about brain death (Veatch, 1983), or even from generic attempts to highlight values as proper parts of medical education because they are inherent in medical practice.

The whole of efforts to incorporate bioethics into policy creation, to render values explicit in public life and evaluate political structures in their light, as in the federal and state ethics commissions now so popular, can be seen as a Deweyan adventure. Bioethics is not only capable of being understood as ethics naturalistically pursued; it is already a naturalism in light of the kind of field it has become since its beginnings in the 1960s.

This last comment requires some elaboration. It may well be argued that the roots of bioethics include some decidedly nonnaturalistic strands, especially the theological ethics that were so important to the beginnings of the field. The important role of theologians and their deontological orientation in the early period is undeniable, but what is noteworthy is that as the field grew in the 1970s, its style and mode of argument became decidedly more empirical or "consequentialist," and theologians and moral theology steadily lost influence. A sociological explanation for this shift might point out that the institutional environment of bioethics changed from small conferences dominated by churchmen in the 1950s and 1960s, to major universities and government panels in the 1970s and 1980s.[3] Without celebrating or bemoaning these historical facts, they can be noted as important forces in the naturalization of bioethics.

3. I owe this insight to John Evans. Personal communication, 1996.

BIOETHICS, AMERICAN SOCIETY, AND DEWEY'S LEGACY

Dewey liked to use the term *social intelligence* in his discussion of the importance of cooperative inquiry conducted in an experimental spirit. At the heart of social intelligence is the use of the best available information to craft improved living conditions. Today we might regard Dewey's call for socially intelligent action as best represented in the policy sciences, wherein a program is implemented according to expressed goals and in light of historic evidence, is evaluated, and then is redesigned in light of actual experience and the extent to which the goals have been achieved. In this respect Dewey and other ethical naturalists resemble the French *philosophes* of the eighteenth century, who arguably founded the notion of public policy.

Bioethicists too operate largely through policy reform and adjustment, whether at the local department or institutional level, or through state or national entities. Even individual interventions—for example, the clinical ethics consultation—are part of a larger effort to enhance the prospects for more general change in the way medical culture deals with ethical issues. The bioethicist is in many respects a policy scientist—or, as some might prefer, a policy humanist.

Dewey's interest in the way values operate in problem solving stemmed from his concern to show that values are not merely abstractions but are crucial in what we might today call policy-making. Dewey thought of values as organizing principles for otherwise undisciplined energies. Values for Dewey were like vectors that galvanize and give shape and direction to energies that must be harnessed for effective social action. The ideas that values have an organizing function and that they have a practical role are perhaps most obvious in a pluralistic society like that of the United States. Anyone who believes that values are not concrete, vital forces has never traversed with open eyes and ears the variegated neighborhoods of a place like Brooklyn.

It is in such a cultural climate that ethical naturalism and bioethics both flourished. In many ways bioethics practices what ethical naturalism preaches. Like the early New World settlers who brought an ancient but abstruse intellectual tradition into the wilderness, bioethicists have by and large been more impressed with what they have found in the clinic than with the philosophies they brought with them. In its attempts to find moral lessons in actual experience—and in its efforts to secure and expand moral values for human enjoyment—bioethics reveals itself as not merely pragmatic but naturalistic.

Among the many fields in which Dewey attempted to apply social intelligence, including education, race and gender relations, disarmament, and industrial policy, medicine would surely have been added to the list if Dewey had lived long enough to witness the technological breakthroughs of the 1960s and 1970s. One philosopher who was strongly influenced by Dewey, Joseph Fletcher, published a pioneering work in which the promises and perils of modern medicine were analyzed from a framework of "situational" ethics (1966), but prior to the full rush of the new biotechnology and without the richness of naturalism as its philosophical background.

Although history did not permit Dewey to become the first bioethicist, it did allow him to articulate a dynamic philosophy that was well suited to American society. America provided fertile ground for the most dramatically new intellectual and social reform movement since the heyday of Continental existentialism and Marxian politics: bioethics.

5

Ethics Consultation as Moral Engagement

What should be the role of the "ethicist" in the clinical setting? In using the term *ethicist,* I am obviously not limiting myself to those who have qualifications in academic philosophy. To do so would be to circumscribe the range of concern too severely, because the qualified academic moral philosopher may often lack other necessary credentials (including the rather nebulous "clinical experience"), whereas the humanistically cultivated healthcare provider may be a competent student of moral philosophy. Moreover, "clinical setting" refers to nursing homes and ambulatory care clinics as well as to hospital in-patient services.

I begin by presenting some doubts about what might be called the "received view" of the role of the moral expert as a healthcare consultant. Then I review the literature on moral experts and moral expertise and proceed to apply the results of that review to the notion that there are some who are expert in ethical decision making in health care. I try to show that certain conclusions that can be drawn from this rather circumscribed topic have implications for the very conception of the relationship between moral theory and clinical ethics.

MORAL EXPERTS IN HEALTH CARE:
THE RECEIVED VIEW

A respected writer and clinical ethics consultant, Terrence F. Ackerman, has articulated the received view of the function of the ethics consultant. The general idea is that the ethics consultant is a "facilitator of moral inquiry" (Ackerman, 1989a; see also 1989b and 1987). For Ackerman this formulation has several implications. First, since moral inquiry is an effort to develop plans for dealing with problematic situations that can evoke a shared social commitment, the determination of morally appropriate behavior requires the contributions of other members of the moral community who participate in reflective moral inquiry. Thus, the ethics consultant cannot simply step in and announce that he or she has "the right answers."

Second, the ethics consultant may nevertheless make recommendations to healthcare providers "about the morally appropriate course of action in a particular situation." These recommendations are founded on the ethicist's belief that these are courses of action that would be endorsed by other reflective members of the moral community. Third, the ethics consultant should facilitate moral investigation by the health professionals themselves. And fourth, the consulting ethicist should be wary of being placed in inappropriate roles, such as those of moral policeman or secular clergyman.

There is much in Ackerman's analysis with which I am in thorough agreement, particularly his emphasis on the role of the moral community. Ultimately, however, this approach fails to come to grips with the true complexity of the ethics consultant's role or the relationship of moral theory to clinical decision making. Among these issues are the theoretical problems with social consensus as a source of authority for moral decision making (Moreno, 1988). More troubling still in the context of Ackerman's formulation is the notion that the ethics consultant's recommendation must square with some imagined result of the moral community's reflection. How is the consultant's belief in this congruence to be sustained? Which moral community is the relevant one? What if the result of that imaginatively projected reflection is itself indecision? Is the ethics consultant no more than a "middle man" between the healthcare providers and the ideal moral community? Must the reflective moral community adopt the same framework of principles as the ethics consultant to be legitimate, or the other way around? Clearly this account cries out for further explanation.

Underlying the received view is the assumption that if only we could get clear on the business of moral expertise it would be a straightforward matter to use the rich resources of moral philosophy to treat tough ethical dilemmas encountered in clinical medicine. In what follows, I will try to show that even a more full-bodied conception of ethical expertise must fall short in the clinical setting unless it is liberated from the prevalent notion that clinical ethics is essentially the application of moral theory to problems in the delivery of health care, or that the role of the clinical ethicist is that of a Socratic "facilitator." I argue that what is required is a substantial reconstruction of the notion of clinical ethics and of our understanding of the ethics consultant's role.

ARE THERE MORAL EXPERTS?

Of the many vexed philosophical problems, whether there are, in fact, moral experts is one issue about which modern philosophers are particularly divided. Though many authors have articulated doctrines that touch on the question of moral expertise, I confine my discussion to some who have addressed it most directly. I begin by presenting two arguments *against* the notion that there can be moral expertise, arguments that tend to crop up frequently in one form or another in the literature.

The first argument is the one that Socrates entertains. It is an argument from analogy with other disciplines to the effect that, since there are recognized experts in other disciplines that most people consider to have something to do with objective matters but none in morality, one has reason to believe that morality is not objective (Burch, 1974). If there is nothing to be objective about, there can be no experts.

The second argument appears in Kant and in another version of Gilbert Ryle: Morality is not the kind of thing in which there can be competence, expert or otherwise, because moral virtue is not a skill. Rather, to be moral is to have a concern for persons, a concern that can obtain as a feature of an individual's character regardless of his or her nonmoral qualities like intelligence or judgment (McConnell, 1984). To think otherwise is to commit a category mistake.

The first, or "no moral experts" view can be countered by showing that the doubt that there are moral experts is unfounded. Often this doubt is characterized by the charge that the advice of so-called moral experts is equivocal. Terrance McConnell (1984) sketches three responses. The first is that moral experts possess general moral principles but not the factual knowledge to apply them; therefore, their expertise is not obvious because its application requires knowledge from two fields, only one of which is within the ethicist's realm of expertise. The second response is that some ethicists do in fact give unequivocal advice. And the third is that experts in other fields also often fail to provide unequivocal answers to problems in which they are supposed to be expert. Moreover, even the presence of conflicting expert opinions or points of view among experts does not distinguish ethics from other fields in which it is generally agreed that there is something to be expert about.

Of these three responses only the first does more than leave open the possibility that there are, in fact, moral experts. The other two have nothing to say about the content of this expertise. A response to the second, or Kant-Ryle argument against the idea that there are moral experts, gives some more detail on this score. Robert W. Burch (1974) contends that the view that morality is a matter of character rather than skill depends on too superficial an understanding of what character is all about. For to the extent that the person of good character is necessarily good at certain things, this will include an ability to discern what is right and wrong and the capacity to be resolute in not taking the easy way out. Moreover, experience suggests that these are not traits that appear ex nihilo; they require a great deal of hard work. The question whether "resoluteness" can properly be considered a matter of expertise is one to which I must return. Finally, that few are in a position to learn from those possessed of these skills can be attributed to the difficulty of the subject as easily as to the nonexistence of its teachers.

These responses to the two arguments against the idea of moral expertise leave us with some ideas about what that expertise might plausibly be like. It involves at least (1) knowledge of general principles and theories of morality, (2) analytic skills such as discernment and insight, and (3) the strength of will not to take the easy way out. Certainly there is room for doubt about each of these elements. Those problems will emerge in the course of examining the implications of this catalogue of elements of moral expertise for the role of the ethicist in health care.

ETHICAL EXPERTISE IN HEALTH CARE

Arthur Caplan (1980) has warned about the limitations of "ethical engineering" in the clinical setting, or the tendency to think that in practice one can provide solutions to troubling ethical issues merely by straightforward deductions from general moral principles. Others, including James Nickel (1988), have called this "strong applied ethics." Elsewhere, Caplan (1983) relates an anecdote that can be used to illustrate the futility of such a scholastic approach. In a situation that appeared to relate to the problem of scarce medical resources, healthcare providers worried that patients with respiratory problems aggravated by summer heat were straining the resources of an emergency room, which had only two oxygen units. Caplan reports that he dutifully consulted the medical ethics texts to see what they had to say about resource allocation. Of course he found not one guideline but various criteria and seemed no better off than the medical staff without the benefit of those theoretical resources. Caplan then asked the staff if Medicare/Medicaid would cover the cost of air conditioners for those afflicted patients, and it was discovered that this was indeed the case, thus "solving" the resource allocation problem.

This anecdote illustrates the limitations of the first substantive qualification for moral expertise in bioethics, knowledge of general principles of morality. In this instance, Caplan knew the principles that could cover the allocation problem, but there were a number of them and none was evidently logically prior or morally superior. Nevertheless, a rigid ethical engineer might simply have selected his or her favorite criterion of distribution and mechanically applied it to the specific problem.

Yet from a different angle, Caplan's solution did exhibit another of the three substantive characteristics of clinical expertise in ethics: discernment. While Caplan's report of this incident is somewhat self-deprecating, the healthcare providers did not come up with his structural question themselves, perhaps because they were too close to the human suffering the problem had engendered. The detachment of the nonprovider on the spot also helps give the discerning disposition a chance to express itself. Caplan also exhibited another of the three proposed characteristics of the ethics expert: he could have taken the easy way out by playing the role of philosopher that the emergency room undoubtedly expected him to play. When he returned with a query about bureaucratic regulations, he risked being seen at least as naïve, at worst as attempting to avoid a tough ethical issue by blaming the problem on financing arrangements.

It could even be argued that Caplan's approach did represent awareness of ethical principles far more basic than those that generated criteria of distribution of scarce resources. In particular, Caplan was surely aware of the principle of equity. It is plausible to suppose that, whether he was fully aware or not, his reluctance to select one criterion over another had something to do with his sense that the results of applying any distribution criterion would not comport as well with this basic ethical principle as a result that treated similarly situated patients in a similar fashion. It is most revealing that his solution accomplished exactly that. Hence, the result was both ethically and strategically satisfactory.

I want to make two observations about the foregoing story. First, in order for the three characteristics of moral expertise I have adduced to be plausible, they must be seen as complementary. Sometimes one characteristic will be more in evidence than another. Second, possession of the first two can confidently be said to depend to some significant degree on formal study of moral philosophy, and I think a good case can be made that while strength of will is not simply or even mainly a matter of education, there is something to the quasi-Socratic, psychological claim that it is hard for people to turn away from what they are rationally persuaded is the right thing to do. Thus, in order for the inclusion of resoluteness on my list of characteristics to be plausible, strength of will must have an ineliminable cognitive dimension.

But why should resoluteness be regarded as a characteristic of expertise per se? Here I want to say that, though it is not strictly a characteristic of expertise, strength of will is a characteristic of the efficacious expert. I take it that this point is undeniable, since those with specialized knowledge who are invited to intervene can hardly be regarded as effective if they sit on their hands for fear of provoking controversy. To the extent that effective intervention is expected of the true expert, irresoluteness will disqualify an individual from such regard.

I have not attempted to "prove" that my list of elements of moral expertise is "correct," though I believe that it captures the elements of other lists of essential characteristics of ethical experts that have been put forward by such philosophers as Peter Singer (1972, 1982). Furthermore, by emphasizing the third quality, strength of will, an additional point is made: the moral expert in the clinical setting often confronts situations in which there is more pressure to "take a stand" than does the moral philosopher in the seminar room. I use the term "take a stand" both in the sense of opposition to institutional routines and pressures, and in the sense of articulating a decisive position.[1] Finally, I believe that this list reflects characteristics that individuals effective as ethicists in health-care settings tend to possess. But this is an empirical claim for which I can as yet offer only anecdotal evidence.

That having been said, there is a final problem about moral expertise in health care that I want to surface, one that I have found troubling in my own experience in an inner-city medical center under enormous social and financial stress. To illustrate

---

1. These proposals, and especially the last, will strike many as Machiavellian. The error lies in a failure to appreciate the depth and significance of the shift from moral philosopher to ethicist, a profound change in role that has in my view been seriously underestimated. But so long as the moral philosopher elects to pursue this new role in the midst of the agora, or a public place like a hospital, the only alternatives to the deliberate acquisition of these skills are blindness to the social complexities of the situation and fumbling efforts to retain academic detachment. If the ethicist in the clinical setting chooses to deny the subtlety of the undertaking by clutching the mantle of moral philosophy, that will rightly be interpreted as arrogance or naiveté. Neither would reflect well on the philosophical traditions that remain our touchstone. An anonymous reviewer pointed this out to me.

this problem I turn again to Caplan's anecdote: it could be argued that his ethical cum bureaucratic solution ultimately helped perpetuate, or at least distract attention from, social arrangements that, in a very general sense, are themselves responsible for the health problems of many poor people.

Now I do not think many would want to take the Leninist position that the present generation should be sacrificed so that the revolution will not be delayed and future generations will benefit. So in its extreme form, this is not a result of healthcare ethics that most want to give up. But there is something to be said for the view that it is a distraction from underlying social problems that clinical ethics enables social institutions to focus on short-term "ethical fixes." Thus we tend to focus on questions such as, "Should all impaired infants be treated?" instead of "Should all pregnant women have access to prenatal care?" "Should drug-addicted pregnant women be incarcerated?" instead of "Should there be enough space in addiction treatment programs for all women of child-bearing age?" and "Should all elderly people be refused certain forms of technological intervention?" instead of "Should there be universal health insurance?" The point is not that all ethical problems result from structural shortcomings, but that concentration on the former distracts attention from the latter.

This criticism of the role of clinical ethics is not directed at ethical experts per se, though one might argue that their presence is an integral part of the distraction. However, I will not pursue this issue. Restated in light of the foregoing, I want to pursue a related charge: that even if the notion of ethical expertise has content, and even if it is not on the whole more detrimental to society than beneficial to have these people participating in "ethics consults" and sitting on ethics committees, there is still something very odd about their role.

TOWARD RECONSTRUCTION IN CLINICAL ETHICS

There are three respects in which the activity of clinical ethics, and therefore the ethicist's role, is crucially different from doing moral philosophy. These differences may be relevant to other forms of the applied philosophy of professional ethics too, so long as it is done in situ; that is, so long as it is conducted with the knowledge that it is likely to affect professional conduct in specific cases.

My purpose is to show that these differences are so important that applied ethics as such—or what Frances Myrna Kamm (1988) has called "*applying* applied ethics"—cannot simply be considered "moral philosophy applied." Because this is not appreciated, there has been no satisfactory analysis of the role of the "bioethicist" or clinical ethicist, whose activities cannot be understood as simply an extension of the traditional role of the moral philosopher. The qualitative difference between moral philosophy and the application of ethics to specific clinical situations in turn imposes different requirements on those who practice in this field. These are large claims that cannot thoroughly be defended here, but perhaps I can at least sketch out the territory relevant to a reconstructed conception of clinical ethics.

There are at least three respects in which moral philosophy and clinical ethics represent qualitatively different activities. First, at the level of practice, since moral philosophers in the Western tradition are suspicious of the moral authority of consensus about moral questions, they are necessarily critics of cultural practices. As a teacher, the moral philosopher has social license to ply this critical trade with students, whose intellectual horizons are thought to be broadened by this encounter. In fact, if moral philosophers do nothing else with their students but take this critical position, calling upon a wide range of learning in the process, then that represents the satisfactory performance of their duties. The Socratic tradition authorizes the critical style as a respectable, if not always constructive, pedagogy.

Now bioethicists are also critics of certain cultural practices, namely, those that have to do with the delivery of health care. They are expected to have insightful and sometimes even unsettling things to say about the way doctors relate to patients or about the priorities evident in current systems of resource allocation and so on. But if the ethicists were *only* critics, they would not be welcome for long in healthcare institutions, but would be derided as inhabitants of an "ivory tower" with nothing helpful to contribute. Rather, ethicists are expected to take a position, give advice, express an educated opinion, or at the very least offer constructive options. This, after all, is the very essence of what it is to be an *applied* ethicist. Again, it is precisely the unwillingness to take a position that is interpreted as lack of resolve in clinical situations, which are not academic and in which some decision must be made.

I am alluding to a familiar experience, even a shocking one, for many philosophers who first make their way around a hospital. As classroom moral philosophers they are allowed to hedge, even expected to do so, but as clinical ethicists this behavior meets with hostility. This is not a trivial difference, for it shows that detachment cannot be the dominant feature of the practice of applied ethics, though it might be for moral philosophy. Again, this difference follows from the different approach to consensus: Western moral philosophy initially requires detachment from received wisdom and permits the philosopher to adopt such an attitude indefinitely; the ethicist, on the other hand, is not permitted to dwell in detachment, but must become engaged.

In reply, it could be said that a sort of Socratic detachment in which moral inquiry is facilitated is and must remain at the heart of what clinical ethics is all about, for this is the unique contribution that philosophers can make to healthcare decision making.[2] But my own experience suggests that the more clinical the context, the less welcome is an exercise that only succeeds in heightening intellectual frustration. Normally, when the ethics consultant is called, the ethical problem is already all too clear to the healthcare providers, and they are in need of a plan of action, sometimes desperately so.

I am not claiming that moral philosophers never become engaged, that they always and unremittingly adopt a critical posture. In fact, this may be true of only a very few of them. My contention is that moral philosophers in their practical role as teachers (and not as authors constructing original arguments), are not *required* to be more than enlightened and enlightening critics (though of course they are often allowed and even encouraged to be more). By contrast, I argue that this is not true of applied

2. This criticism I owe to Edmund Pelligrino.

ethicists in the clinical setting, who *are* required to be more than critics. At the other extreme, the danger that engagement will turn ethicists into preaching moralists is met only insofar as the ethicist is prepared always to re-evaluate his or her own views, and this involves adopting the critical posture again.

The second important reason that clinical ethics cannot simply be understood as moral philosophy applied has to do with the historic development of the great moral theories. Bioethics, particularly as it was finding its philosophical feet in the 1970s, has frequently adopted a methodology that entailed the following steps: coming across a "hard case" in which ordinary "common sense" yielded inconclusive moral intuitions; reaching for an important moral theory or two, usually some version of Kantianism and consequentialism; and applying the theories to the hard case. If the theories yielded the same results, one could at least be satisfied with this commonality; but if the theories yielded different results, one was thrown back on theoretical justification. Since the latter is not a bioethical but a moral philosophical task, the bioethicist's choice of a solution often had an arbitrary air.

More importantly, the recognition that the above methodology would not always yield satisfactory results in terms of the hard cases undermined confidence in the moral philosophies themselves. Around this time important philosophers, especially Alasdair MacIntyre (1981) and Richard Rorty (1979) presented forceful anti-foundational arguments. MacIntyre's approach, in particular, emphasized the conflicts between systems of moral discourse around hard cases like abortion.

In my view, this way of thinking about moral philosophies, broadly understood, rests on a misunderstanding, and the assessment of a moral philosophy or form of moral life should not rest solely, or even mainly, on its treatment of the so-called "hard case." One reason for this is that the great moral philosophies were not designed to address specific conceptual dilemmas, but to create panoramic views of the good life, the "great-souled human being," the just society, or the right mode of conduct. The instances in which those philosophies in their classical expressions do tackle specific cases have not generally been regarded as their finest hours: recall Kant's application of his moral philosophy to the problem of telling the truth about someone's whereabouts in the presence of an enemy bent on murder. While it is of course possible to derive standards, guidelines, or criteria from them, the theories are usually rich enough to admit various interpretations: consider, for example, the familiar difficulties in deciding which of several alternatives "maximizes utility" even after all the data is in. It is true that the hard case helps chart the limits of a system of moral belief, but because it stimulates the moral theory to express its richness, the exercise often produces ambiguous and therefore ultimately unsatisfying results.

For the clinical ethicist, moral theory provides some orientation, but only in a broad and general sense, for it can also prove disorienting once the various theories' multiple implications for the hard case are discerned, as they will be when the theory is used to throw light on some particular case. Thus, again, applied moral philosophy is not simply moral philosophy applied. Clinical ethics is like a river with many tributaries, and moral philosophy is only one, though major, tributary.

A hackneyed response to the realization that there is no royal road to bioethical truth through moral theory is that "there are no answers," a refrain heard more often in the 1970s when the approach described was more common. But the point is that moral philosophy cannot in itself provide "the answers," or at least not in the genuinely hard cases, and I think there is a reason for this in addition to the one I have just discussed.

The hard cases are such precisely because they reveal the points at which systems of moral belief rub up against each other. In homogeneous societies, the limits of the belief systems may not be noticed or may not engender great public controversy; but in pluralistic societies such as ours, "the answers" must satisfy constituents of moral points of view that differ, though these differences are often only at the edges. Because the differences are so intractable, they tend to exaggerate the contrasts between the moral theories.

In such a situation, the ethicist is in a position to do more than teach, criticize, and analyze. Because he or she is conversant with the nature of moral belief in a general sense, the ethicist is well-placed to discern hitherto unrecognized ways in which rival belief systems might be "stretched" (e.g., the adult child who wants "everything done" for her parent with multiple system failure but will consent to a do-not-resuscitate order to avoid vegetative existence); or reasonably modified (e.g., the surgeon who agrees to delay a risky corrective procedure for a heart defect in an infant with numerous uncorrectable anomalies in order to assess the child's pulmonary potential); or even defensibly constrained (e.g., the practice of obtaining court orders to transfuse children of Jehovah's Witnesses). As the ethicist becomes more directly engaged in this process, he or she assumes a role in the "political" processes that are an essential part of the management of rivalries among communal values.

Beyond a certain point it is useless to wonder whether the clinical ethicist should participate in these processes or not. As soon as the individual identified as the "moral expert" leaves the seminar room or library for the hospital conference room or nursing station—that is, when the moral philosopher no longer trades only in theory and hypothesis but participates in institutional decision making about particular cases—the transformation from moral philosopher to ethicist has been accomplished. In these circumstances the clinical ethicist must adopt the sanguine posture that the moral philosopher's intellectual abilities can be brought to bear, but not without some further skills required of participants in human institutions. Thus the outstanding question is, what skills besides moral expertise does the ethicist require? While this question invites a study in itself, I will close with some brief suggestions.

It is often said that the nonphysician ethicist must be familiar with the language of health care in order to be effective. But there are at least three other sorts of skills that are required for ethicists to play their inherently political role effectively. Probably they all suggest a level of formal training that few ethicists, if any, can claim, but it would be surprising if the best clinical ethicists did not have sound intuitions in these directions. First, the ethicist should be a skilled participant-observer, able to identify informal social structures and arrangements and to assess his or her developing role in them. Second, the ethicist should understand the dynamics of small group behavior, with an ability to recognize the interplay between sociometric structures and decisional outcomes. Third, the ethicist should be a competent mediator, familiar with negotiating strategies and having sound interpersonal skills.[3] Taken together, the development of educational programs to impart these skills represents a significant challenge for clinical ethics.

3. Ackerman (1987) reaches similar conclusions. The difference between us is the significance each of us attributes to the fact that these personal skills are substantial departures from those normally required of the moral philosopher.

6

Ethics by Committee:
The Moral Authority of Consensus

A survey of eighteen hospital ethics committees asked the respondents to indicate their method for identifying when a decision has been reached. Of the eight respondents who directly answered that question, all mentioned consensus. Virtually all the rest described their procedures in a way that left the impression that consensus was the method (Cranford and Doudera, 1984). Similarly, a report by several members of an ethics committee concerning their procedures identifies "unanimity or consensus" as the preferable closure.

While a substantial literature has emerged concerning the alternatives for operating these committees—their legal status, composition, and institutional roles and responsibilities (e.g., Cranford and Doudera, 1984; Fost and Cranford, 1985; Kliegman et al., 1986; Lynn, 1984; Robertson, 1984)—virtually no attention has been given to the development of a "consensus ethics" that has come to be these committees' conclusory standard. Yet for bodies engaged in the articulation and application of moral principles in health care, it is obvious that the adoption of a consensus model has ethical implications of its own. What, then, is the moral significance of consensus? In this chapter I adopt a more approachable paraphrase of this question: What is the source of moral authority in an ethics committee that operates by means of consensus?

To answer this question, I want to develop a philosophical framework for the consensus-oriented ethics committee. First, I consider the actual functions of these committees in a healthcare bureaucracy, paying special attention to their problems, limitations, and dangers. Second, I briefly set out a well-known dilemma in moral epistemology about moral truth in general, an ontological debate with practical consequences for ethics committee deliberations. Next I formulate guidelines for committee functioning in terms of what might be called "vertical" and "horizontal" dimensions: comparison of the crucial features of cases and review of arguments for degrees of their plausibility. Then I note the different levels of consensus for which ethics committees may strive. After placing the notion of committee deliberation in the context of two liberal political theories, I conclude that the idea of consensus should be thought of primarily as a *condition* of deliberation rather than its goal. I believe that this corrects a mistake at the heart of the confusion about consensus.

Throughout this chapter it will be necessary to shift back and forth between philosophical analysis and the demands of realpolitik, that is, the ethics committee's setting. This is because the ethics committee stands at the muddy intersection of ethics in theory and in practice, rendering a philosophical framework all the more elusive and important.

I do not concern myself here with other forms of ethical consultation that take place outside a committee or group setting. Nor do I distinguish between ethics committees concerned with the care of infants and those concerned with adults, since the consensus standard appears to be prevalent regardless of the patient population involved.

ETHICS COMMITTEES AS COMMITTEES

In the trivial sense that they represent bureaucratic lines of authority and control, all committees are political entities. It is therefore no wonder that ethics committees have adopted the standard of consensus, for like autonomy, consensus is a political concept that has been imported to ethical territory. But unlike the concept of autonomy, consensus has not yet undergone systematic and intense scrutiny in medical ethics. Much can be learned from sociologists who distinguish between consensus by "head count" and by acquiescence (e.g., Stanley, 1978), or who study patterns of small group interaction (e.g., Simmel, 1950). Whether their conclusions are optional or mandatory, and whether they review or make policy, we need to know what moral weight to ascribe to committee positions. This will require greater theoretical and empirical examination of the actual operation of consensus.

Some contend that due to their inherently political nature committees can never be more than reflections of established powers, poor sites for resolving an institution's moral quandaries (Lo, 1987). Certainly, a committee system can easily lead to abuse, since members may be held in thrall by the authorities who have appointed them. I am not prepared to concede that for purposes of ethical consultation committees are necessarily corrupt, though their nature warrants caution (Levine, 1984; Siegler, 1986). Later in this essay I will suggest that sound procedures are the best protection against abuse.

It might be argued that there is no interesting difference between an ethics committee and any other bureaucratic entity in a complex social structure like a hospital. What distinguishes it is not its multidisciplinary membership, its procedures, or its political or legal functions, all of which might be similar to other committees. Rather, according to this view, the only difference is that the content of its issues is, or is supposed to be, specifically ethical in nature. These issues merely fall into one category of medical practice and administration, a category for which a certain sort of committee is established. In the hospital management scheme, the ethics committee fills a niche parallel to those filled by many others. Thus, one could argue, there is no reason that consensus should not close discussion in ethics committees as it may for any committee operating in and for the institution. On this view a simple majority would be definitive were it not for the odd notion that ethics should not be a matter of majority rule (when hardheaded social observers tell us that it often is).

Moreover, the actual work of many of these bodies does not always consist in helping resolve ethical disputes as a moral philosopher or theologian would understand that term. Indeed, addressing communication problems, searching for further facts, or uncovering medico-legal misconceptions are among the activities typical of ethics committees. The diverse and often contentious activity of ethics committees has been described elsewhere (Macklin, 1988). Even when genuinely ethical issues arise, often the committee's task is to identify the authoritative literature and apply its conclusions. Paradoxically, ethics committees do not always, or even usually, worry over ethical dilemmas. This state of affairs is less surprising when it is recalled that the term was popularized through the *Quinlan* decision by a judge who was actually talking about prognosis committees (Weir, 1987).

Yet there are at least two good reasons to worry about the moral authority of consensus in ethics committees. First, some of these committees do find themselves asked to comment on hard cases or institutional policy options involving conflicts of moral values. Second, merely because of their name, ethics committees will often be seen as lending a special kind of authority to their advice, even if the content of the advice is not, strictly speaking, about a moral dilemma.

The potential for the ethics committee to be perceived as a unique authority in a hospital is apparent in another way. Unlike other committees in an institution, the ethics committee may in principle reasonably withdraw from a case without being viewed as having abdicated its responsibilities. For if no solution acceptable to all parties seems available, the committee may take the position that it would be inappropriate for it to force a particular point of view in a morally vague area. To do so would leave the impression that it is reasonable to force a single committee's ethical consensus on everyone else.

An ethics committee's withdrawal from a controversy would effectively leave the problem to an administrative or legal remedy. In fact, most committees stress an "advisory" rather than a "decision-making" capacity, regarding their functions as mediation and the improvement of communication. As though to emphasize this, some committees do not even call themselves committees but use some less suggestive title such as "group" or "forum." This characteristic also partly distinguishes the present-day ethics committee from other bodies in the history of medical decision making that have performed tasks with ethical implications, for example, kidney dialysis allocation committees (Alexander, 1977). It would have been far more difficult for those other entities to withdraw from a controversy and retain their status in the institution.

CONSENSUS AND ETHICAL EXPERTISE

Medicine is a consensus-driven system. That is, the practice of consultation among experts relies on a standard of intersubjective agreement, as is true of any practice that relies on scientific generalizations implicitly viewed as warranted. In an area like medicine, where objective information is often inconclusive regarding particular cases, consensus has an explicit role. But of all the committees in the healthcare institution, only the ethics committee appears to be as consensus-oriented. One reason for this may be a widespread sense that it is unseemly to "settle" ethical questions by a mere vote. Another may be intensely practical: there is simply no way to impose an ethical view on hospital personnel unless there is broad agreement among those who are widely perceived to be representative of various units. Perhaps most importantly, the ethics committee operates on the borders between patient care and hospital management. The consensus approach is borrowed from the former, and the committee concept from the latter. The patient care/consensus approach gives experience and expert judgment special importance in the committee.

This is not the place to rehearse those fundamental issues of moral epistemology that underlie problems of authority and knowledge in ethics. Intuitionist, rationalist, and naturalist approaches to the evaluation of moral reflection interact with various views about the influence and propriety of social ideals and sanctions (Foot, 1967). Admitting the superficiality of mere reference to these problems, at least one should be leery of the notion of expertise in determining what counts as a morally correct course of action, especially since the content of that expertise is still a matter of debate (Caplan, 1983). This is one reason that the very idea of an "ethics committee" frequently meets with warranted resistance.

Related to the problematic nature of expertise are deep philosophical doubts about the practical possibility of consensus. In recent years there has been a celebrated line of argument to the effect that the modern social world is so constituted that only an illusory agreement about matters related to cultural values is possible. Alasdair MacIntyre's *After Virtue* (1981) is a pointed rejection of the prospects of moral agreement in the modern West. On epistemological and linguistic grounds, MacIntyre holds that the Babel of valuational tongues we have inherited from multiple cultural traditions renders our moral discourse impotent. A case in point is that classical—and classically recalcitrant—struggle, the abortion debate.

MacIntyre is surely correct that substantive values may not be sharable or even meaningful across cultural boundaries. There may nevertheless be procedures that help lead to agreement for purposes of action. Later I will argue that those procedures can be discerned in the process of ethical deliberation itself.

MacIntyre's reintroduction of a virtue ethic helps to explain why some physicians resist ethics committees: ethics consultation seems subversive of the doctor's claims to personal morality. Though apparently less prevalent now than in the early days of clinical biomedical ethics, some physicians still construe questions about their decision making as veiled attacks on their own moral character. A virtue ethic is subtly inculcated in traditional medical education. For in this tradition, ethical medicine is best ensured by morally good doctors, while effective medicine is protected by consultation among technical experts that yields consensus.

This attitude has recently softened, giving way to the ethics consult as merely another relevant perspective in the development of a treatment plan, and the ethics committee as merely another sort of mechanism to review or secure professional consensus. In this way ethical questions have been drawn into the system of expert consensus, so much so that there has been little attention paid to philosophical reservations about institutionalizing moral guidance through group structures. This is surprising, because the history of Western philosophy is replete with warnings about the special danger of permitting individuals to cede moral responsibility to groups. As has been noted, modern social psychology is full of accounts of this distortion of rational decision making by the effects of small group interaction. A single strong personality can exercise undue influence over others, for example. The consensus can be a cover behind which hide timidity, lethargy, self-interest, and even social pathology (Lo, 1987).

Still, it is hard to see how any standard other than consensus could prevail in the—at least officially—anti-authoritarian social setting in which contemporary health care functions. Ultimately, I believe, this is one of a range of problems with consensus that will continue to seem insoluble so long as consensus is regarded primarily as a goal rather than as a condition of ethical deliberation.

CONSENSUS AS CONSTITUTIVE OR EVIDENTIARY

Consensus is important in medicine because of uncertainty both at the level of biomedical theory and at the level of application of theory to some particular cases. Where there is scientific uncertainty but action must be taken, agreement among experts may legitimately rely on gut feelings or "clinical experience." Presumably, if one were to query physicians about the epistemological significance of their educated guesses, the vast majority would turn out to be realists. That is, they would tend to believe that the agreement of those with a great deal of clinical experience is evidence that the independently correct answer is being approximated. On this view, authoritative consensus has evidentiary force. Of course, it would be entirely consistent, though culturally rare, for a practitioner to reply that a certain level of intersubjective agreement actually constitutes the truth. Instead of thinking of the biomedical community as discovering the truth about some technical aspect of medicine, this respondent would think of the community as cooperating in the creation of that truth, more or less.

Perhaps the point can best be made by imagining that an epistemological realist and a non-realist are colleagues on an ethics committee. The non-realist assumes that any consensus that is regarded as authoritative—by whatever standards—will be the truth of the matter. On the other hand, his or her realist colleague expects a morally authoritative consensus—again, by whatever standards—to approximate and perhaps even discover the truth of the matter, a truth that is independent of the consensus itself (Daniels, 1986).

Notice that for each there can be such a thing as consensus. For the constitutive non-realist, true consensus is achieved only if all rational considerations that are relevant to the case at hand have been taken into account. These rational considerations could also tend to counteract those irrational or irrelevant considerations that have seeped into these deliberations. Unless this condition is met, the consensus will last only until those neglected rational considerations can no longer be ignored.

The evidentiary realist in moral theory operates according to criteria familiar to realists in the philosophy of science (Pierce, 1955). A true consensus is one in which the various shades of opinion tend to converge or cohere. A false consensus is one in which they seem to converge but, on closer examination, are perceived to diverge and even contradict. With regard to her own views, the evidentiary realist is a fallibilist, prepared to admit that any views she holds may turn out not to be approximations of the truth of the matter, which she is nevertheless confident does exist.

The nature of realism in moral epistemology has been well rehearsed elsewhere (Railton, 1986). I am inclined to agree with those philosophers who have derided all debates about realism as spurious (Rorty, 1983). But I will pursue that point later.

The subject of realism versus non-realism is introduced in order to make the point that one can devise a formal check on the ethics committee process regardless of where one falls on this issue. As a general recommendation, on this line of reasoning an ethics committee wishing to conduct a retrospective review of its own advisory opinions or decisions should be guided by both tests used in a complementary fashion. It could ask, first, whether any rational considerations have been excluded, systematically or otherwise, in this case. Second, it could ask whether the opinions tend to converge into a more or less coherent pattern. This dual approach could cover both of the seemingly opposing bases in the debate between moral realism and non-realism.

This puzzle about what ethics committees ultimately do is a springboard to a better understanding of their process. From this epistemological dispute it is possible to gather some good questions that any ethics committee that has dealt with an ethical dilemma in a case or policy should ask itself.

For many ethics committees there may be too small a body of cases to generalize about, particularly if the actions taken on individual cases usually involve resolving problems of communication rather than substantive ethical dilemmas. Moreover, committees engaged in shaping policy recommendations for their institution, such as those involving patient or family requests for termination of treatment, will have to modify the dual test proposed above according to the answers to the following: Have all rational considerations been weighed concerning this matter of moral controversy? Have views converged such that a coherent approach to the problem is available?

Admittedly, this double-barreled check on moral deliberation could lead to more rather than less ethical uncertainty. For the more rational considerations that are weighed, the less convergence may be forthcoming. Or the greater the apparent convergence of opinions, the greater the temptation to set aside some arguably rational considerations. Philosophically, these conflicts could be taken to refer to the unresolved tension between realism and non-realism or to the incoherence of the problem. Procedurally, they could be seen as features of a full and open airing of the issues in an atmosphere of self-consciousness about the process itself.

It is worthwhile to be aware of the relevance of this philosophical debate about realism to the idea of consensus. Finally, however, I will argue that to approach consensus in terms of this debate is misguided, and that whatever the merit of ethics committees is, it cannot be grounded in this conceptual framework. To see why an alternative framework is needed, I will now consider the conceptual levels at which consensus may play a role in these bodies.

LEVELS OF CONSENSUS

When they do address cases or policies that engage ethical dilemmas properly so called, ethics committees rely on consensus primarily because of the unsettled nature of the issues. These issues may involve either ethical ambiguity or ethical conflict. The former occurs when some interpretation of the underlying relevant ethical principles is required, for there is lack of clarity about the proper application of the principles to the present case or the policy being proposed, but there is no apparent disagreement about the rightness of the principles themselves. This sort of dilemma involves disagreement about the rightness of the way the principles have been brought to bear on this case or proposed policy. Thus, in one instance, what is required of the committee is consensus about application of principles, while in the second instance what is required is consensus about principles, or "deep consensus."

It is important to distinguish between these two sorts of consensus because agreement at one level does not guarantee agreement at the other. Ethics committee deliberation may not go so deep as the discussion of the merit of principles themselves; indeed, my experience is that striving for deep consensus is quite exceptional. Rather, what is routine is the effort to reach consensus at the level of cases *simpliciter*. Reactions and intuitions are exchanged by committee members following a review of medical, psychosocial, and legal factors. Rarely are underlying values questioned, except perhaps by a philosopher or theologian who happens to be a committee member. Stephen Toulmin, citing his own experience as a consultant and staff member with the National Commission for the Protection of Human Subjects of Biomedical and Behavioral Research, reports that disagreements about principles themselves were infrequent; more divisive were views about how to apply certain principles or what principles should be used to reach a conclusion about which there was agreement. The differences among the commissioners did not reveal themselves until each gave "reasons" for his or her conclusion. Toulmin explains this phenomenon by appeal to the nature of the deliberations on the "hard cases" up for review: "They inquired what particular conflicts of claim or interest were exemplified in them, and they usually ended by balancing off those claims in very similar ways" (Toulmin, 1986).

Toulmin's experience is surely familiar to those of us who have participated in similar deliberations. We may find ourselves in a group that reaches more or less the same conclusion for different reasons. Those differences can be the result of interpreting or weighing the same principles somewhat differently or can arise from selecting entirely different principles that happen in this instance to lead to the same conclusion. From this Toulmin draws the lesson that attention to cases allows the degree of certitude appropriate to practical reasoning in ethics, an important point that I will elaborate and clarify in the next section. Ultimately, I will come back to a still deeper lesson to be learned here: that for moral deliberation to proceed in this manner, certain conditions must be obtained.

Upon reflection on Toulmin's remarks, there is room for a particular worry: does it follow that the members of an ethics committee might be better off not to examine too closely their reasons for taking one view or another, lest they discover the depth of their differences and compromise their ability to function together? Then how can the committee be sure that its decisions are well-founded, if the results of group self-consciousness about principled differences are so threatening that self-study is avoided?

This conundrum does not necessarily represent either a defect in the idea of the ethics committee or an escape from moral or intellectual responsibility on the part of committee members. It does suggest that closer theoretical attention must be paid to whatever wisdom inheres in the form of deliberation on cases or policies in ethics committees.

Indeed, it seems likely that straightforward conflicts of basic values are rare, so broad and bland are those values. Thus we may agree in general that "respect for life" is a basic ethical principle yet discover that we interpret it or balance it against other values quite differently. Some philosophers would say that in that case we do not really hold the same idea at all (Rorty, 1961). Leaving the epistemological problem aside, it is clear that even when a number of people believe that the idea to which they assent is the same, there is no guarantee that action will be uniform. In a given case, the ethics committee could identify the hitherto unrecognized competing values and weigh those values as they are found in this case as compared to their roles in others. Again, it appears that attention to the nature of deliberation itself is important.

ARGUMENT AND COMPARISON

In the following analysis of the form of ethical deliberation in a committee setting I will be both prescriptive and descriptive. I will cite some successful models of two methods of ethical deliberation, methods that I believe should be complementary in ethics committees when they deal with ethical issues. I do not underestimate the importance of empirical information about group process, but I think it is fair to say that there are some guidelines that have proven their worth.

One method of deliberation is familiar. It is a disciplined approach to a moral problem that can generate arguments of varying degrees of plausibility. I call this the *vertical method,* because of the implicit reference to a hierarchy of admissible arguments. When policy formation is the aim, the vertical method is sufficient. The other method places the present case on a continuum of settled cases and sorts out the present ethical dilemma through comparison. This *horizontal method,* though less familiar than the other, in fact has a long and venerable history in the tradition of casuistry.

As my example of the vertical method I will use the review of arguments regarding the withholding and withdrawing of life support in the President's Commission report on decisions to forgo life-sustaining treatment (1983a). There the Commission had already depreciated the distinction between action and omission, or even its tenability in specific instances. Nevertheless, it recognized a view that the withdrawal of a treatment must meet a higher standard of justification than withholding. The argument in support of this view is that if withdrawing a treatment is causally related to a patient's death, this constitutes (actively) killing the patient, whereas not starting it is an act of omission that "merely" lets the patients die. In response, the authors observe that the line between withdrawing and withholding is often hard to draw, so the distinction is unreliable in principle. The example given involves a power failure during the use of a respirator: does the decision not to use a manual bellows count as withholding or withdrawing treatment? It is suggested that proponents may save the moral significance of the distinction between withholding or withdrawing by referring to the patient's expectations of continued treatment that may be created by the initiation of therapy. However, the Commission notes that discussion between a patient and physician may alter the patient's expectations. Moreover, the view that treatment once initiated can never cease can indirectly have lethal consequences, since it may cause physicians not to try a therapy that might be of benefit to the patient because they fear that there will be no way to stop it.

These arguments are well known. I repeat them in this context only to use the pattern of argument as an example of a familiar, disciplined approach to an ethical issue, part of the dialectical tradition. A thesis is propounded and supported by an argument; qualifications and counter-examples are presented in response; the thesis is further defended by reference to principles and/or consequences; it is shown that the principles need not be violated nor need the consequences follow; and the coup de grace shows a far more serious compromise of principles and/or consequences that follow from the original claim. Furthermore, when this model of a disciplined review of arguments is circulated in a report of this kind, its substantive results can be used by a committee as a background against which to test the arguments of, say, a particular clinician on a similar question. Thus, it can undertake its own review of arguments informed by that in the Commission's report. The Socratic dialogues are examples of the pursuit of this form of deliberation as a group process. Gradually, more and less acceptable arguments can be viewed along a hierarchy of dialectical adequacy.

A complementary horizontal method is one that has all but disappeared in name but not in practice. For the past century, the casuistic tradition has been more criticized than understood, but Albert Jonsen (1986) and Stephen Toulmin (1988) provide a reconstruction of casuistry that is relevant to a style of moral deliberation that is still popular (see also Murray, 1987).

Casuists worked from cases, setting them out in a way that showed the connection between a kind of case and a certain principle. Ordinarily the connection is probabilistic, for there is no direct relation between the theoretical principles of moral theory and the practical principles of morality. Yet the moral theory is essential background for the practice, just as medical science is essential to prevent the practice of medicine from degenerating into quackery (Jonsen and Toulmin, 1988). What is therefore sought in normative moral judgment is rational agreement about the likelihood that a particular conclusion is correct.

Casuists would thus take an authoritative definition of an important term such as "killing" and arrange a number of cases from the clearest instances to the progressively less-clear instances of killing. Working from the paradigm case, they would search for those variations that turn out to be critical in the determination that some cases did instance killing. They would also seek the maxims in a case, those unquestioned moral principles that are not further demonstrated but help to develop a moral argument. Examples of such maxims are "Don't kick a man when he is down" and "One good turn deserves another," the sorts of guiding principles of morality that ordinary people use in conversation. Other features of casuistic method adumbrated by Jonsen and Toulmin include the addition of complicating circumstances and, finally, the assessment of the probability of a conclusion.

It was the richness of its method that got high casuistry into trouble and led to subsequent negative associations with the term. So many variations were introduced that the product resembled moral philosophy's version of the system of Ptolemaic epicycles. But upon reflection, it is striking how much of the deliberation in contemporary biomedical ethics is unconsciously casuistic: assembling an array of cases, searching for the decisive points of comparison, and identifying morally relevant differences. For example, it is now common to regard treatment decisions for severely ill newborns as falling along a continuum, from those who should certainly be treated to those for whom treatment should be forgone. Down syndrome infants with a surgically correctable physical defect would be at one end and anencephalics at the other, while infants born with a meningomyelocele or trisomy 18 or 13 would be among those occupying various positions in between. This continuum may appear obvious now, but in fact it was the result of a difficult debate that began well before the Bloomington Baby Doe (Duff and Campbell, 1973).

When ethics committees deal with a case rather than a policy, they might array the present case against other clearer cases and proceed by means of comparison, contrast, and analogy. Those cases could be found in a variety of sources, from casebooks to those in the committee's experience. If I am correct that a great deal of casuistic reasoning takes place in ethics committee deliberations, it would be useful to learn in more detail about the casuistic method and to apply it more systematically.

Having these complementary deliberative methods in hand, it becomes somewhat harder to appreciate the force of the problem with consensus. After all, they have both been used in what are commonly regarded as instances of bioethical deliberation that have yielded authentic conceptual advances. If the methodology is sound, then as in any process of inquiry, that methodological soundness will help to authorize confidence in results achieved through its use. I believe that this is an important point, one that I will be able to elaborate after laying some groundwork borrowed from social philosophy.

CONSENSUS RECONSIDERED

Given these complementary methods of moral deliberation, a major remaining question is whether and why the multidisciplinary membership so commonly thought to be important for ethics committees has any philosophical merit. It is not difficult to understand the political importance of having a broad spectrum of units represented on a committee that deals with sensitive subject matter. It is also sensible to have information from various fields when the subject matter is likely to have many dimensions. But is there any more general philosophical importance to breadth of membership? I believe that there is, that it is a key to the moral authority of consensus understood primarily as a condition of deliberation in ethics committees, and that it cannot be divorced from the needs for political representation and specialized knowledge. At the end of this path will be an alternative account of the nature of consensus itself.

A naïve view of the desirability of broad representation on an ethics committee leads to a variety of confusions about the nature of ethical consensus as well. That view takes representation in the sense relevant to a legislature. Thus, the point is to gather members of various affected constituencies—doctors, nurses, social workers, administrators, lawyers, chaplains, ethicists—and ascertain whether some controversy can be settled in a way that would be satisfactory for each constituency. It would be advisable to include representatives of the patient population as well (a good practice in any case, in my experience).

This view of the ethics committee as a kind of legislature is incoherent. First, it suggests that some democratic process is required for the selection of members, otherwise the legislature is likely to be a House of Lords, selected by administrative authorities. (We would probably have to ask the mayor or city council to select the patient representatives). Second, if it is a mini-legislature, then majority rule is as good as consensus, and certainly more efficient. The result of all this is that ethical dilemmas reduce to political controversies without a trace of residue.

The liberal tradition that provides the framework of our secular society offers two typical accounts that are improvements over this inadequate version of the moral significance of representation. I will refer to these accounts by way of the writings of H. Tristram Englehardt Jr. (1986) and John Dewey (1929, 1935). I take Englehardt to be an example of a libertarian or "right liberal" social philosophy, while Dewey can be regarded as a "left liberal." Their crucial common feature, that which places them both firmly within the Western liberal tradition, is their commitment to personal autonomy. But from there they diverge.

Englehardt's bioethical theory presupposes conflict. Because it is unlikely that any particular conception of the moral life will be decisive, it is necessary to establish a procedural basis for ethics. This procedural basis Englehardt finds "in the very nature of ethics itself," that of "peaceable negotiation among the parties to a controversy." This minimum condition of ethics also delivers what

Englehardt regards as a necessary condition: "the requirement to respect the freedom of the participants in a moral controversy." The protagonists must respect one another's autonomy as the basis for all further interaction or else power rather than reasoned discourse will "settle" the issue (Englehardt, 1986).

For Englehardt, since ethical discussion begins as conflict among parties with deeply held conceptions of the moral life, it is vital to respect those differences. Seen in this light, an ethics committee can help ensure that various points of view are recognized and appreciated, and whatever proposals emerge should be respectful of the liberties of the groups represented. The point of the representation is to ensure respect for those rights that are enjoyed by various affected constituencies. These rights or liberties can be moral as well as legal; therefore, the committee does not simply replicate a court of law.

This right liberal view of the ethics committee that I have inferred from Englehardt's bioethical theory has much to recommend it. In particular, it places the ethics committee "movement" within the framework of the dominant thrust of contemporary biomedical ethics, that of protecting the right of patients to determine the course of their own treatment. I suppose that on this view a case would not even come before an ethics committee without the autonomous patient's request for consultation. Presumably, an ethics committee could also protect certain professional rights, insofar as they do not clash with those of the person who is actually to be treated.

It is tempting to criticize this view as a minimalist ethics that is narrowly fixated on limiting interference with freedom of action. But like John Stuart Mill, Englehardt is careful to insist that societies may create any positive form of social life they like so long as they do not violate the basic requirements of liberty (Mill, 1975). Consensus is required to certify that no one regards any of those forms as such a violation. Therefore, the premise is that social organization must be constrained from violating liberties in the negative sense of "freedom from" interference, and this is more basic than the promotion of liberty in the positive sense of "freedom to."

To identify what is wanting in this approach, one must focus on its Hobbesian picture of social life: any sort of controversy can easily degenerate into a war of all against all; therefore, let us guard against brutality by enshrining a doctrine of mutual respect. But one may doubt that many of the problematic situations that arise in life, moral or otherwise, are matters of such profound controversy that they threaten to throw us into some primeval social jungle. The burden of this claim falls on the Hobbesian. What seems far more typical is that questions are cooperatively resolved, at least temporarily, according to some more or less systematic method. Rather than viewing cooperation as a possibility that might also emerge from social life, the right liberal sees a method of reasoned inquiry as imposed on a recalcitrant natural order, threatening always to break down.

By contrast, the left liberal regards cooperative deliberation as a systematic method that emerges from natural conditions themselves, so cooperation is at least as "natural" as dispute. Moreover, individuality is seen, not as an atomistic state to be jealously defended, but as a precondition for consummatory experience that must be nurtured. To assume otherwise is to suppose, among other things, that each individual has an essential nature logically prior to society, a dualism that carries a great deal of dubious ontological baggage. Calling his the method of "social intelligence," Dewey holds that inquiry begins with a problematic situation and that liberty must be guaranteed or else all deliberation is at hazard.

Like the right liberal, Dewey regards freedom as a condition for social action, an instrument in the construction of social goods, but he does not regard it as the only fit goal of sociopolitical activity. To Dewey, freedom from interference in the pursuit of goods is not necessarily the basic role of social organization, which may also be obligated—on the ground of preserving or promoting freedom—to create forms that help individuals to attain concrete goods. The very distinction between "negative" and "positive" freedom is specious, on this view. The semantic distinction "freedom from" and "freedom to" often makes no practical difference and should not take precedence over the protection of the individual's opportunity for participation in the consummatory experiences that social organization has made possible. The limitations of right liberalism are well summed up in Dewey's words: "The thing which now dampens liberal ardor and paralyzes its efforts is the conception that liberty and development of individuality as ends exclude the use of organized social effort as means" (Dewey, 1935, 90).

It remains for cooperative inquiry to identify desirable goals of human activity and set out to achieve them, sometimes altering a notion of that which is desirable during the project. The massive achievements of the sciences, including, of course, the biomedical sciences, Dewey took to be paradigmatic for all other areas of inquiry, ethics included.

If ethics committees are seen as sites for the exercise of social intelligence, a number of their qualities can be thrown into relief. Professional expertise is crucial for intelligent deliberation, and like any inquiry that requires information and techniques from various disciplines, the group must be composed to fill those requirements. Members are gathered to lend their abilities to the clarification of a problematic situation in which each field has something to contribute, including the experience of being a patient.

I am now in a position to make my view of consensus clear. Ordinarily, it seems, consensus is regarded as a goal to be reached. I contend that this puts the cart before the horse. The point of ethical deliberation is not to reach consensus but to attain a desirable end, an end that settles a controversy without further disagreement. Along the way there must be agreement about the soundness of the method being used. Thus, consensus is not an abstract end. It conditions a process of cooperative reconstruction of a troubling situation into one in which whatever latent values there are can be recognized and, by taking some action, perhaps more fully enjoyed. The way in which this is proposed to be done is an hypothesis, subject to change in light of attempts to apply it.

Perhaps a specific case example will help with the last point. An 85-year-old woman has suffered a number of strokes and has been placed on a respirator. The recommendation for a do-not-resuscitate order has been rejected by her daughter, who had not seen the patient for a number of years prior to her current illness. The physicians and nurses believe that cardiopulmonary resuscitation would be burdensome and futile for the patient, whose wishes are unclear.

Both the right and left liberal approaches would take as critical the interest of the patient not to have useless and burdensome treatment imposed upon her. But since it is not obvious that this is her desire, the right liberal approach seems hampered by the inability to identify a right respecting which would protect the patient's autonomy. The alternative approach I have outlined can take into account other latent values in the situation; thus, I believe it is more in tune with the subtleties inherent in actual situations of ethical uncertainty. An ethics committee consulted in this situation might note, for example, that a final reconciliation between the daughter and her mother might end the daughter's reluctance to approve of an order, facilitate communication that clarifies the patient's wishes, and enable both to gain an experience of intrinsic value in resolving years of alienation. Thus, it could urge the caregivers to cooperate with social workers in moving toward this goal, rather than insisting upon an immediate order.

I do not mean to suggest that particular situations are always clear, nor that they allow a clear distinction between the two approaches. I introduce this example to illustrate the differences in the way a committee might operate: as the guardian of a patient's rights with other factors as at best secondary concerns, or as the promoter of goods consistent with that of the patient's right. As practiced by an ethics committee, the method of social intelligence recognizes that ethically troubling situations express an interplay of possibilities. To make the best of a bad bargain is to retrieve and enlarge upon whatever goods are available. Once again, consensus is a condition of that aim, not an end in itself. To put it another way, consensus refers primarily to the process of moral deliberation in groups of human beings and only derivatively to the conclusion that is reached.

It would, of course, be entirely possible for consensus per se to be identified as the goal of a committee deliberation. But this would be a very odd and unsatisfactory state of affairs: "I don't care what you decide," someone in authority says to the ethics committee chair, "just so you all agree!" Yet this is what is implicit in the notion that committees "strive for consensus." Surely, what they strive for is a morally satisfactory result reached through a cooperative, open, and rational method in which all have expressed persistent confidence through their participation.

Finally, I want to observe that this model of social intelligence is especially compatible with the two methods of deliberation I described earlier. The disciplined approach to the evaluation of arguments brings intelligence to bear in much the same manner as does the testing of an hypothesis. (The patient's wishes are unclear, and reconciliation is desirable; perhaps both can be satisfied with a little more time). In seeking the maxims in a case, casuistic method attempts to identify its inherent values. (In the case mentioned, the relevant maxim might turn out to be "Let bygones be bygones"). Dewey himself frequently refers to the importance of maxims and proverbs in the appreciation of the values that are part of the fabric of human experience.

CONCLUSION

I have argued that those ethics committees that deal with issues of ethical uncertainty can profit from understanding both their peculiar status in an institution and the philosophical problems of knowledge in ethics. I have also claimed that there are complementary methods for moral deliberation that can be of value to ethics committees in light of the problems associated with different levels of consensus. And finally, I have urged that a Deweyan social philosophy would recast the notion of consensus altogether as primarily a condition of cooperative ethical deliberation rather than as an end in itself.

PART THREE

HUMAN USE

Introduction

I can't say exactly when I was captured by issues in human research ethics. They weren't the problems that I started with, nor are they for other students of bioethics, who tend to worry first about the seemingly more immediate concerns described in Part One. Whenever it was, I was struck by the unavoidable and seemingly irresolvable exquisite moral framework of clinical research: that it involves using a person as a means to someone else's benefit, and does so while applying and refining what are among the most impressive expressions of humanity: ingeniously crafted scientific ideas.

Nearly as soon as I acquired an appreciation for the richness of this framework, I was also struck by the richness of the history of research involving people and by how difficult it can be to identify circumstances that satisfy the diverse moral requirements of ethical research. As a philosophical naturalist, I often find myself exploring both of these topics in the same discussion, and each of the chapters in this section more or less reflects that approach. They are also all characterized by a preoccupation with measures to protect people who participate in research. Considering that advancing science is, and ought to be, seen as generally a good thing, this preoccupation makes little sense without a strong historical sensibility.

Another point I try to make here is that the notion enshrined in current federal regulations that certain groups require *special* protections is incoherent without access to the historic record. That is, it's obviously not a necessary fact of history that children or prisoners have been disproportionately used in medical experiments, but it is contingently true, based on the facts. On the other hand, what does seem inescapable is that being institutionalized does increase the chances that one will be used in research, and since institutionalization is associated with lessened self-determination, justice demands that any such groups receive special consideration when experiments are proposed.

It was, in fact, the lack of historical justification that led me to resign as publicly as I could from the Bush administration's advisory committee on human research protections in January 2003. I had been appointed to the equivalent committee by the Clinton administration, but the charter of that panel was allowed to lapse in mid-2002. The Bush administration then re-wrote the committee's charter to include "embryos" as one of the vulnerable groups about which it would advise the Secretary of the Department of Health and Human Services. But embryos have never been the subject of public discussion as to whether they should be added to the list of vulnerable groups (pregnant women and their fetuses, prisoners, and children), and I objected to what seemed to me to be the obvious politicization of a science advisory committee charter. When the administration's sloppy staff work then led me to be one of only three people to be reappointed to the new committee, I took the opportunity in the press to announce that I would not serve. It is the only time I have ever felt it was better not to be on the inside. I also complained that no one from a patient's advocacy group was on the new panel, and I was pleased that one was appointed to take my place.

Finally, if any additional population should in theory be included in special research protections, it should be those who lack decision-making capacity, like people with advanced Alzheimer's.

There are complex historical reasons for this failure of our regulatory scheme, but there is also the practical problems of determining who among those at risk for impaired decisional capacity need some extra protection, and exactly what form those protections should take. I wrestled with this problem as a consultant to the National Bioethics Advisory Commission in 1998, when I was responsible for drafting the NBAC report on this subject. After a good ten years of thinking about it, this is a set of issues about which I remain particularly unsettled.

7

Goodbye to All That: The End of Moderate
Protectionism in Human Subjects Research

A NEW WORLD ORDER

In May 2000 the Secretary of the Department of Health and Human Services announced new regulatory and legislative initiatives concerning federally sponsored research involving human subjects. Around that time, the Office for Protection from Research Risks (OPRR) was reconstituted as the Office for Human Research Protections (OHRP) and, with a new director, completed its transition to the Office of the Secretary, Department of Health and Human Services (HHS). Both the OPRR and the Food and Drug Administration (FDA) had been increasingly active in sanctioning institutions with malfunctioning ethics review boards and those that had engaged in questionable research practices, especially in human genetics trials.

Weeks after HHS Secretary Donna Shalala's announcement, a bipartisan group of congressional sponsors led by Congresswoman Diane DeGette (D-CO) introduced the Human Research Subjects Protections Act of 2000. Among other reforms, the Act would extend informed consent and prior review requirements to all human subjects research, regardless of funding source. Senator Ted Kennedy (D-MA) introduced a bill that would establish steep civil penalties for investigators and institutions that broke the rules. Leading up to all this activity were several congressional hearings on the subject since 1997 as well as numerous reports and recommendations by public and private panels concerning the state of the regulatory system.

All these hearings, bills, and reports had one thing in common: they all found or presupposed a need to strengthen the human subjects protections system. Although some individuals representing the community of scientific investigators raised their voices in objection to increased regulation—especially the psychiatric community in response to the National Bioethics Advisory Commission's recommendations concerning research involving persons with mental disorders—theirs were largely voices in the wilderness. Protests that new measures would block important research seemed hard to sustain in light of two decades of remarkable advances under the current system, which, at the time of its introduction, was itself predicted to be so burdensome as to threaten new medical breakthroughs. Reservations about increased bureaucracy, or even the question whether the proposals being advanced would have avoided any actual patient or subject injuries, were overwhelmed by a historical tide that presages a new era in the history of human subjects regulations, an era that I call *strong protectionism*.

The essence of strong protectionism is the minimization of clinical researchers' discretion in governing their conduct with regard to human subjects. Among the measures implied by strong protectionism are concurrent third-party monitoring of consent and study procedures, disclosure of financial arrangements or other potential conflicts of interest, required training of investigators in research ethics and research regulations, and independent review of the decision-making capacity of potential subjects. All these and other measures have been proposed, and many of them may be implemented in spite of the additional costs in time and money they represent and regardless of the inference an observer may draw that clinical researchers are simply not to be trusted.

In this chapter my purpose is neither to challenge nor defend these early stirrings of what I believe to be a new era in the history of human subjects protections. It is, rather, to note how inured we have become to this grim view of investigator discretion and how far we have traveled to reach this pass. The current transition to strong protectionism builds upon a singularly important period of about thirty-five years, from 1947 to 1981. That period witnessed the breakdown of an ancient tradition of *weak protectionism* that granted enormous discretion to physician experimenters. What followed was an era that is currently passing away, a compromise between physician discretion and modest external oversight that I call *moderate protectionism.*

Perhaps it was inevitable that moderate protectionism could last only about twenty years. It was a compromise that combined substantial researcher discretion with rules enforced by a minimal bureaucracy. An important part of this compromise was that researchers for the most part had the prerogative of identifying potential conflicts of interest themselves, without external review. Researchers' use of human subjects was approved before and after it actually took place, but (with a very few institutional exceptions) not during research activities themselves.

The moderately protectionist era might have lasted longer had the research environment not changed so much, had so much money not poured into research as the result of promising new areas for investigation and investment, had the proportion of private funding not increased so drastically, and had the number and complexity of studies not grown so rapidly. Together, all these elements stressed the twenty-year compromise called moderate protectionism, perhaps fatally, even though it was a period little blemished by harms to persons, at least as compared with the scandalous era that immediately preceded it.

WEAK PROTECTIONISM: VIRTUE HAS ITS DAY

Concerns about the involvement of human beings in research are at least a century old. Many institutionalized children were subjects in vaccine experiments in the nineteenth century both in Europe and the United States, and by the 1890s anti-vivisectionists were calling for laws to protect children. At the turn of the century the Prussian government imposed research rules, and Congress considered banning medical experiments for certain populations such as pregnant women in the District of Columbia. In the ensuing decades there were occasional well-publicized scandals, mostly involving child subjects, and the first attempt to test a polio vaccine was stopped after the American Public Health Association censured the program (Lederer and Grodin, 1994).

Prior to the Second World War, however, medical researchers were largely inoculated against regulation by the nearly legendary status of the self-experimentation by members of U.S. Army physician Walter Reed's Yellow Fever Commission in Cuba. One of the commissioners, Dr. Jesse Lezear, died after subjecting himself to the mosquito's bite, helping to confirm the hypothesis of the disease's spread. A less celebrated but equally notable element of the Reed story is his use of an early written contract for the Spanish workers who were among the commission's other subjects, which itself appears to have followed a controversy involving yellow fever research subjects (Lederer, 1995).

For some reason Reed himself was widely thought to have been one of the volunteer subjects, perhaps due to his untimely death only a few years later that resulted from a colleague's error. This misconception added to the legend and to the model of medical researchers as of exceptional moral character, even to the point of martyrdom. The Reed mythology became a singular reference point and justification for the self-regulation of medical science. During the 1960s, when researchers were coming under new levels of scrutiny and weak protectionism was under attack, the distinguished physician-scientist Walsh McDermott referred to the Reed story to demonstrate the social importance of research and the high moral standing that went with it (McDermott, 1967).

Thus, by the early 1950s, although there were gestures in the direction of a protectionist attitude toward human subjects, even these expressions were in a fairly abstract philosophical vein rather than in a robust set of institutionalized policies and procedures. An example is the army's failure to implement a compensation program for prisoners injured in malaria or hepatitis studies when it was contemplated in the late 1940s (ACHRE, 1996). The essential feature of the weak form of protectionism that prevailed at that time was its nearly wholesale reliance on the judgment and virtue of the individual researcher. Reflecting the medical community's dissatisfaction with the legalistic tone of the Nuremberg Code, deliberations on the World Medical Association's Helsinki Declaration of 1964 (Helsinki I) began in 1953. Informed consent was a far less prominent feature of the first Helsinki Declaration than of the Code. Helsinki also introduced the notion of surrogate consent, permitting research when individuals are no longer competent to provide consent themselves. These moves place a substantial burden on the self-control of the individual researcher, a point to which I shall return (Faden and Beauchamp, 1986).

To be sure, until the middle and later 1960s, and with the significant exception of the Nazi experience, to many there did not seem to be good reason for worries about human protections. The development of penicillin, the conquest of polio, and the emergence of new medical devices and procedures apparently unmarked by inappropriate conduct all bolstered the public prestige of biomedical research. Nevertheless, there were some inklings of a continuing, albeit low-intensity, concern about the concentrated power of medical researchers even in the 1950s, exemplified perhaps in the gradual disappearance from professional discussions of the term "human experiment" and its replacement with the more detached and reassuring term "research."

On the whole, then, the world of clinical studies from the late 1940s through the mid-1960s was one in which a weak form of protectionism prevailed, one defined by the placement of responsibility upon the individual researcher. Written informed consent (through forms generally labeled "permits," "releases," or "waivers"), though apparently well-established in surgery and radiology, was not a common practice in clinical research; and in any case, it cannot be said to have provided more than a modicum of increased protection to human subjects. For example, whether a medical intervention was an "experiment" or not, and therefore whether it fell into a specific moral category that required an enhanced consent process, was a judgment largely left up to the researcher. Partly that judgment depended on whether the individual was a sick patient or a healthy volunteer. The former were as likely as not to be judged as wholly under the supervision of the treating doctor even when the intervention was quite novel and unlikely to be of direct benefit. Therefore, an individual might be asked to consent to surgery but not be informed beyond some generalities about its experimental aspect.

There were, however, some important exceptions. For example, the Atomic Energy Commission established a set of conditions for the distribution of radioisotopes to be used with human subjects, including the creation of local committees to review proposals for radiation-related projects. Early institutional review boards were established in several hospitals (including those at Beth Israel in Boston and the City of Hope in California) to provide prior group review for a variety of clinical studies. Another exception seems to have been the Clinical Center of the National Institutes of Health in Bethesda, Maryland, which opened in 1953. A government-supported research hospital, the Clinical Center appears to have been one of a handful of hospitals that required prospective review of clinical research proposals by a group of colleagues.

As advanced as the Clinical Center might have been in this respect, the prior group review process it established seems, at least at first, to have been confined to healthy, normal volunteers. The moral equivalence of at least some sick patients who would probably not be helped by study participation, to normal subjects who would not be benefited (with the possible exception of vaccine studies) was apparently not appreciated in policy. These subtleties were largely lost in a period in which medical discretion and societal benefit weighed heavily.

Prior group review, which is essential to the transition beyond weak protectionism, was not common before the 1970s. Yet decades earlier there was a keen awareness of the psychological vulnerability inherent in the subject role, a vulnerability that could have argued for independent review of a research project. An extensive psychological literature, founded mainly on psychoanalytic theory, propounded a skeptical view of the underlying motivations of experiment volunteers as early as 1954. That year Louis Lasagna and John M. Von Felsinger reported in *Science* on the results of Rorschach studies and psychological interviews of fifty-six healthy young male volunteers in drug research. The authors concluded that the subjects exhibited "an unusually high incidence of severe psychological maladjustment." "There is little question," they wrote, "that most of the subjects . . . would qualify as deviant, regardless of the diagnostic label affixed to them by examining psychiatrists or clinical psychologists." The authors theorized that this group may not have been representative of the population from which it was drawn (college students), and that they might have been attracted to the study for various reasons having to do with their deviance, beyond financial reward (Lasagna and Von Felsinger, 1972).

I describe this study, not to endorse its psychology or its conclusions, nor to imply that neurotic tendencies are either typical of research volunteers nor a priori disqualifying conditions for decision-making capacity. The point is, rather, that as early as 1954 thought was being given to the question of the recruitment of subjects who might be vulnerable despite their healthy and normal appearance. The article was published in a major scientific journal. It would have been natural to ask further questions about the vulnerability of potential research subjects known to be seriously ill. Yet despite this psychological theorizing, which could be viewed as quite damning to the moral basis of the human research enterprise, protectionism was at best a weak force for years to come.

DOUBTS TRIUMPHANT

An occasion for the significant revision of this picture became available at the end of the Second World War, when twenty-three Nazi doctors and medical bureaucrats were tried for crimes associated with vicious medical experiments on concentration camp prisoners. The defendants were selected from about 350 candidates. Although only 1,750 victims were named in the indictment, they were only a handful of the thousands of prisoners used in a wide variety of vicious experiments, many in connection with the Nazi war effort. Some involved the treatment of battlefield injuries or prevention of the noxious effects of high altitude flight. Others, such as the sterilization experiments, were undertaken in the service of Nazi racial ideology, and still another category had to do with developing efficient methods of killing.

A strong defense mounted by the defendants' lawyers pointed to the fact that the Allies too had engaged in medical experiments in the service of the war effort. As the prosecution's attempt to demonstrate that there were clear international rules governing human experimentation faltered, the judges decided to create their own set of rules, known to posterity as the Nuremberg Code, the first line of which is: "The voluntary consent of the human subject is absolutely essential." Although the court seemed to believe that protections were needed, it is not clear how intrusive they wished these protections to be in the operations of medical science. The judges declined, for example, to identify persons with mental disorders as in need of special provisions, although urged to do so by their medical expert. The very requirement of *voluntary* consent for all undermined the relevance of their code to experiments involving persons with diminished or limited competence, and the extreme circumstances that gave rise to the trial itself seemed quite distant from normal medical research (Moreno, 1999).

Unlike the medical profession as a whole, the new Atomic Energy Commission in 1947 apparently took note of the Nazi doctors' trial and attempted to impose what it termed "informed consent" on its contractors as a condition for receiving radioisotopes for research purposes. It also established—or attempted to establish—a requirement of potential benefit for the subject. Both of these conditions were to apply to nonclassified research. This relatively protectionist attitude may not have been adopted with a great deal of appreciation of its implications. In any case, the AEC's position met with resistance among some of its physician contractors but not its physician advisors. The AEC's early protectionist stance finally did not become institutionalized, and the letters setting out the requirements seem to have soon been forgotten. (The potential benefit requirement seems itself to have been incompatible with all the trace-level radiation research the AEC sponsored shortly thereafter.) Similarly, in the early 1950s the Department of Defense adopted the Nuremberg Code, along with written and signed consent, as its policy for defensive research on atomic, biological, and chemical weapons; but a 1975

Army Inspector General report pronounced that initiative a failure (ACHRE, 1996).

Historians of research ethics generally date the increasing vigor of protectionist sentiment among high-level research administrators and the general public to the series of events that began with the Thalidomide tragedy and continued with scandals such as the Brooklyn Jewish Chronic Disease Hospital case and later the Willowbrook hepatitis research. These cases cast doubt on the wisdom of leaving judgments about research participation to the researchers' discretion. The Jewish Chronic Disease Hospital case, in which elderly debilitated patients were injected with cancer cells, apparently without their knowledge or consent, was one of those that attracted the attention and concern of the National Institutes of Health's director, James S. Shannon. Shannon's intervention, and the resistance from within his own staff, was an important and revealing moment in the history of human subjects protections.

In late 1963 Shannon appointed his associate chief for program development, Robert B. Livingston, as chair of a committee to review the standards for consent and requirements of NIH-funded centers concerning their procedures. The Livingston Committee affirmed the risks to public confidence in research that would result from more cases like that of the Jewish Chronic Disease Hospital. Nonetheless, in its 1964 report to Shannon, the committee declined to recommend a code of standards for acceptable research at the NIH on the grounds that such measures would "inhibit, delay, or distort the carrying out of clinical research." Deferring to investigator discretion, the Livingston Committee concluded that NIH was "not in a position to shape the educational foundations of medical ethics" (ACHRE, 1996).

Disappointed but undeterred by the response of his committee, Shannon and Surgeon General Luther Terry proposed to the National Advisory Health Council that the NIH should take responsibility for formal controls on investigators. The NAHC essentially endorsed this view and resolved that human subjects research should only be supported by the Public Health Service if "the judgment of the investigator is subject to prior review by his institutional associates to assure an independent determination of the protection of the rights and welfare of the individual or individuals involved, of the appropriateness of the methods used to secure informed consent, and of the risks and potential medical benefits of the investigation" (Reisman, 1965). The following year Surgeon General Terry issued the first federal policy statement that required PHS-grantee research institutions to establish what were subsequently called Research Ethics Committees (Curran, 1970). The seemingly innocent endorsement of "prior review by institutional associates" was the most significant single departure from the weakly protectionist tradition, leading to a process that finally yielded the moderately protectionist system we have today.

The Surgeon General's policy was, however, hardly typical of contemporary attitudes, and the practice it sought to implement is one we are still trying to effect. To appreciate the weakness of the form of protectionism that prevailed through the 1960s, it is useful to recall the dominant role that prison research once had in drug development in the United States. By 1974 the Pharmaceutical Manufacturers Association estimated that about 70 percent of approved drugs had been through prison research. Pharmaceutical companies literally built research hospitals on prison grounds. Although in retrospect we may think of modern limits on prison research as a triumph of protectionism (on the grounds that prisoners cannot give free consent), at the time it was a confluence of political and cultural forces that had little to do with actual abuses (though there certainly were some), and these reforms were resisted by prison advocates. Perhaps the most important public event that signaled the inevitable end of widespread prison research was the 1973 publication of "Experiments behind Bars" by Jessica Mitford in the *Atlantic Monthly*.

Within the medical profession itself, then, weak protectionism remained the presumptive moral position well into the 1970s, if not later. Neither of the most important formal statements of research ethics, the Nuremberg Code and the Helsinki Declaration, had nearly as much effect on the profession as a 1966 *New England Journal of Medicine* paper by Harvard anesthesiologist Dr. Henry Beecher. The importance of timing is evident in the fact that Beecher had been calling attention to research ethics abuses since at least 1959, when he published a paper entitled "Experimentation in Man," but his 1966 publication "Ethics and Clinical Research" attracted far more attention. One important distinguishing feature of the latter work was Beecher's allusion to nearly two dozen cases of studies alleged to be unethical that had appeared in the published literature. By "naming names" Beecher had dramatically raised the stakes.

It would be an error, however, to conclude that Beecher himself favored external review of clinical trials that would remove them from medical discretion. To the contrary, Beecher was one among a large number of commentators who favored (and in some instances continue to favor) reliance primarily upon the virtue of the investigator. Although he strongly defended the subject's right to voluntary consent, he argued in his 1959 paper that "an understanding of the various aspects of the problem" being studied was the best protection for the human subject, and he was quite critical of the Nuremberg Code's dictum that the subjects themselves should have sufficient knowledge of the experiment before agreeing to participate.

Beecher's attitude toward the Code's provisions was hardly limited to philosophical musings. In 1961 the army attached Article 51, which was essentially a restatement of the Nuremberg Code, to its standard research contract. Along with other members of Harvard Medical School's Administrative Board, Beecher protested and persuaded the Army Surgeon General to insert into Harvard's research contracts that its Article 51 were "guidelines" rather than "rigid rules" (ACHRE, 1996).

Beecher's attitude was shared by many other distinguished commentators on research practices through the 1960s and 1970s. In 1967 Walsh McDermott expressed grave doubt that the "irreconcilable conflict" between the "individual good" and the "social good" to be derived from medical research could be resolved, and certainly not by "institutional forms" and "group effort"—apparently references to ethics codes and peer review. McDermott's comments were by way of introduction to a colloquium at the annual meetings of the American College of Physicians on "The Changing Mores of Biomedical Research." In his remarks, McDermott alluded to the growing contribution of research to the control of disease, beginning with Walter Reed's yellow fever studies. Thus, he continued, "medicine has given to society the case for its rights in the continuation of clinical investigation," and "playing God" is an unavoidable responsibility, presumably one to be shouldered by clinical investigators (McDermott, 1967).

Another distinguished scientist who made no secret of his skepticism toward the notion that the investigator's discretion could be supplemented by third parties was Louis Lasagna. In 1971 Lasagna wondered "how many of medicine's greatest advances might have been delayed or prevented by the rigid application of some currently proposed principles to research at large." Rather, "for the ethical, experienced investigator no laws are needed and for the unscrupulous incompetent no laws will help" (Lasagna, 1971: 105). Six years later, the National Commission for the Protection of Human Subjects of Biomedical and Behavioral Research proposed a moratorium on prison research. In a caustic response, Lasagna editorialized that the recommendations "illustrate beautifully how well-intentioned desires to protect prisoners can lead otherwise intelligent people to destroy properly performed research that scrupulously involves informed consent and full explanation and avoid coercion to the satisfaction of all but the most tunnel-visioned doctrinaire" (Lasagna, 1977: 2349).

It is perhaps worth noting that both Beecher and Lasagna had good reason to reflect on the problem of research ethics, stemming from some work they did together. Between 1952 and 1954 Louis Lasagna had been a research assistant in a secret army-sponsored project, directed by Beecher, in which hallucinogens were administered to healthy volunteers without their full knowledge or consent. Recalling the episode in a 1994 interview with the President's Advisory Committee on Human Radiation Experiments, Lasagna reflected "not with pride" on the study (Lasagna, 1994).

WEAK PROTECTIONISM: THE DEATH KNELL

Among those who developed an interest in research ethics during the 1960s was Princeton theologian Paul Ramsey. Although Ramsey is today remembered as one who took a relatively hard line on research protections and he did in fact significantly advance the intellectual respectability of a protectionist stance, in retrospect his position seems remarkably modest. In his landmark 1970 work *The Patient as Person,* Ramsey declared that "no man is good enough to experiment upon another without his consent" (Ramsey, 1970, 7). In order to avoid the morally untenable treatment of the person as a mere means, the human subject must be a partner in the research enterprise. However, Ramsey was prepared to accept nonconsented treatment in an emergency, including experimental treatment that might save life or limb. He also acceded to the view that children who cannot be helped by standard treatment may be experimental subjects if the research is related to their treatment and if the parent consents.

The emergence of modern bioethics at the end of the 1960s brought another nonphysician commentator, Hans Jonas, onto the scene. While generally agreeing with the theologian Ramsey in advocating strict limits on professional discretion, the philosopher Jonas struck a more passionate, even haunting tone: "We can never rest comfortably in the belief that the soil from which our satisfactions sprout is not watered with the blood of martyrs. But a troubled conscience compels us, the undeserving beneficiaries, to ask: Who is to be martyred? in the service of what cause? and by whose choice?" (Jonas, 1972: 735). In explicitly calling forth survivor guilt among those who benefit from the sacrifices of experimental subjects, Jonas also deepened the moral burden on the clinical investigator and called attention to the moral paradox of human experimentation.

By 1970 the notion that consent was ethically required was well established in principle (including surrogate consent for children and incompetents); however, it was poorly executed in practice. Ramsey's contribution was in calling attention to the problem of *nonbeneficial* research participation, a decision that required at a minimum the human subject's active participation, while Jonas nevertheless insisted on the inherent and unavoidable unfairness of all human experimentation. As though to underline the point, only two years after Ramsey's and Jonas's writings, the Tuskegee Syphilis Study scandal, a case in which the subjects were clearly not informed participants in the research and were used as mere means, broke into the open. The federal review panel appointed to review the study, the Tuskegee Syphilis Study Ad Hoc Panel, concluded that penicillin therapy should have been made available to the participants by 1953. The panel also recommended that Congress create a federal panel to regulate federally sponsored research on human subjects, a recommendation that foreshadowed and helped to define the later transition from weak to moderate protectionism.

A casualty of the syphilis study was the attitude exemplified in the 1967 essay of Walsh McDermott and the 1969 paper by Louis Lasagna. In the years immediately following Beecher's 1966 article it was still possible to argue that scientists should take responsibility to make what McDermott regarded as appropriately paternalistic decisions for the public good, decisions that recognize that societal interests sometimes take precedence over those of the individual. Although there clearly are instances in which this general proposition is unobjectionable, following the syphilis study such an argument became much harder to endorse in the case of human experiments. In a word, the tide of history was turning against the physician commentators, who were united in their defense of a system based on the responsible individual investigator.

As the implications of the Tuskegee revelations became apparent, philosopher Alan Donagan published an essay on informed consent in 1977 that symbolized the altered attitude. Donagan's critique ventured well beyond those of Ramsey and Jonas, which were written before the Tuskegee revelation. In Donagan's essay the invigorated informed consent requirement is taken as nearly a self-evident moral obligation in clinical medicine. In his discussion of informed consent in experimentation, Donagan explicitly compared the arguments of a Nazi defense attorney with those of McDermott and Lasagna, concluding that they are both versions of a familiar and, one infers, a rather primitive form of utilitarianism. Donagan concluded that by the lights of the medical profession itself the utilitarian attitudes instanced in the Nazi experiments and the Brooklyn Jewish Chronic Diseases Hospital case cannot be justified. Perhaps still more telling about the evolution of the moral consensus concerning research ethics is the mere fact that Donagan, a highly respected moral philosopher who could not be dismissed as a "zealot," could associate the arguments of Nazis with those of some of America's most highly regarded physicians. Donagan's essay underlined a leap in the evolution of protectionism through the Tuskegee experience, especially on the question of the balance between the subject's interests and those of science and the public, and on the subsequent discretion to be granted the lone investigator (Donagan, 1977).

TWO FORMS OF ACCESSIONISM

To be sure, the story I have to tell is not one of an inexorable march toward a stronger form of protectionism, even in the past twenty years. Although the tendency since the advent of the Nuremberg Code—greatly strengthened in the United States by the Belmont Report—has been to limit the scope of investigator discretion, there have been countervailing forces. One of these has been the Declaration of Helsinki, which uses the concepts of therapeutic and nontherapeutic research, defining the former as "Medical Research Combined with Professional Care." According to Helsinki IV (1989), "If the physician considers it essential not to obtain informed consent, the specific reasons for this proposal should be stated in the experimental protocol for transmission to the independent committee." Thus Helsinki continues to contemplate a relatively permissive attitude toward investigator discretion, as it has since the first version in 1954. Notably, Henry Beecher preferred Helsinki to Nuremberg precisely because the former is a "set of guides," while the latter "presents a set of legalistic demands" (Refshauge, 1977).

Another force counteracting the tendency to limit investigator discretion has been movement on behalf of greater access to clinical trials. The most pronounced expression of this effort has occurred among AIDS activists, who successfully insisted on the creation of alternative pathways for anti-AIDS drugs in the late 1980s. In the face of a disease that resisted treatment and struck down people just entering the prime of life, the determination to find solutions was understandable. The slogan of ACT-UP (AIDS Coalition to Unleash Power) that "A Drug Trial is Health Care

Too," was a political expression of confidence in the power of science. As well, the slogan betrayed assumptions about the benefits of research participation and the self-discipline of the medical research community, relying on the very protections it sought to undermine. It should be said that activist organizations have largely revised their attitude toward alternative pathways of access to nonvalidated medications. This movement might be called *therapeutic accessionism.*

In contrast to therapeutic accessionism, there has been another and far longer lasting movement on behalf of *scientific accessionism.* In the late 1980s female political leaders noted the paucity of women in clinical trials, leading finally to significant changes in NIH and FDA policies. Similarly, policy reforms have recently been introduced for children. Unlike therapeutic accessionism, this view seems likely to persist and is, in fact, consistent with the Belmont Report's principle of justice as it attempts to further extend the benefits of research. Also unlike the earlier position taken by some AIDS activists, the call for greater participation in clinical trials by women and children is wholly consistent with strengthened protections.

BEYOND MODERATION

Arguably, moderate protectionism was being dismantled as soon as it was born. In the early 1980s the President's Commission for the Study of Ethical Problems in Medicine and Biomedical and Behavioral Research made recommendations on the evaluation and monitoring of institutional review board (IRB) performance (1983b) and also endorsed the proposition that research-related injuries should be compensated (1982). The impact of the President's Commission's efforts to sustain the pressure brought to bear by the National Commission for the Protection of Human Subjects was muted, however, by a relatively (and uncharacteristically) scandal-free period in the history of human research ethics. Instead, the pressing needs for new medications in the wake of the AIDS epidemic, and the accessionist movement that went with it, was dominant for much of the 1980s and early 1990s.

The serenity was challenged in the 1990s by the revelations of cold war radiation experiments. Though they took place decades before, the human radiation experiments story provided an occasion for another look at the regulatory regime and how well it was working. Among the recommendations of the Advisory Committee on Human Radiation Experiments in 1995 were several that would strengthen human subject protections. For example, the ACHRE urged that regulations be established to cover the conduct of research with institutionalized children and that guidelines be developed to cover research involving adults with questionable competence. The ACHRE also recommended steps to improve existing protections for military personnel concerning human subject research. Substantial improvements were urged in the federal oversight of research involving human subjects: that outcomes and performance should be evaluated beyond audits for cause and paperwork review; that sanctions for violations of human subjects protections be reviewed for their appropriateness in light of the seriousness of with what the nation takes failures to respect the rights and welfare of human subjects; and that human subjects protections be extended to nonfederally funded research. The ACHRE also recommended that a mechanism be created for compensating those injured in the course of participation as subjects of federally funded research (ACHRE, 1996).

Within eighteen months of the ACHRE's final report, on May 17, 1997, the National Bioethics Advisory Commission unanimously adopted a resolution that "no person in the United States should be enrolled in research without the twin protections of informed consent by an authorized person and independent review of the risks and benefits of the research" (NBAC, 1997). That same month President Bill Clinton stated, "We must never allow our citizens to be unwitting guinea pigs in scientific experiments that put them at risk without their consent and full knowledge" (Clinton, 1997). At the end of 1998 the NBAC recommended increased protections for persons with mental disorders that might affect their decision-making capacity, reminiscent of suggestions made by the National Commission twenty years before (NBAC, 1998). On the whole, two decades since its advent, moderate protectionism was on the run before a flurry of federal activity.

WHITHER PROTECTIONISM?

On the account I have presented, protectionism is the view that a duty is owed those who participate as subjects in medical research. The underlying problem is how to resolve the tension between individual interests and scientific progress, where the latter is justified in terms of benefits to future individuals. Weak protectionism is the view that this problem is best resolved through the judgment of virtuous scientists. Moderate protectionism accepts the importance of personal virtue but does not find it sufficient. Strong protectionism is disinclined to rely, to any substantial degree, on the virtue of scientific investigators for purposes of subject protection. We are today so accustomed to moderate protectionism that we have nearly forgotten the struggle that led to its establishment. Where once it was considered radical, moderate protectionism is now embraced by the medical community. Consider, for example, the position exemplified in a recent essay on ethics in psychiatric research in which the authors state that "the justification for research on human subjects is that society's benefit from the research sufficiently exceeds the risks to study participants." But then the authors continue, "Potential risks and benefits must be effectively communicated so that potential subjects can make informed decisions about participation" (Lieberman et al., 1999, 25). The current battleground, then, is not whether the subjects should in theory be full participants, or whether prior review of experiment proposals should be required, but whether, or to what extent, subjects can take an active role in the clinical trials process. To the extent that such active participation can be achieved, the introduction of more strongly protectionist requirements may be forestalled.

Implicit in all discussions about the ethics of clinical trials has been the assumption that the investigator bears a significant degree of moral responsibility for the dignity and well-being of the human subject, a responsibility that cannot be sloughed off and assigned to someone else. In the words of the first article of the Nuremberg Code,

> The duty and responsibility for ascertaining the quality of the consent rest upon each individual who initiates, directs or engages in

the experiment. It is a personal duty and responsibility which may not be delegated to another with impunity.

This sensibility has not wholly disappeared from our public discourse, even in the onslaught of calls for higher levels of subject protection by regulatory means. Rather, the dispute turns on how much we should rely on the moral virtue of the individual investigator. While he was still a medical school professor, the person who would later be the first director of the Office for Human Research Protections wrote a passage explicitly reminiscent of Beecher's sympathy for a system based on the scientist's virtue. "In truth," wrote Greg Koski in 1999, "investigators are much better positioned during the course of their studies to protect the interests of individual research subjects than are the IRBs. Paradoxically, the person most likely to do something to harm a subject, the investigator, is also the person most capable of preventing such harm. And so, as Beecher (1966) concluded many years ago, the only true protection afforded research subjects comes from a well-trained, well-meaning investigator" (Koski, 1999, 225).

Koski's admiration for Beecher (another Harvard anesthesiologist) is evident, but his peroration has an air of nostalgia about it. Certainly, following his assent to the OHRP directorship, Koski did not return to this sentiment, at least in his public statements, but joined the historic march toward more protectionist arrangements.

A MORAL HAZARD

I have argued that the march of history is resolute in its rejection of the investigator discretion articulated by the Nuremberg judges, later advocated by Beecher, and recently recalled by Koski. There is nonetheless a moral hazard in the strong protectionism that aims to supplant the scientist's virtue.

It would be understandable, if not admirable, were the assumption about the scientist's personal responsibility for his other subjects to be undermined among future clinical investigators operating in a much more intensely regulated environment. Paradoxically, the research scientist's sense of personal moral responsibility might weaken as the official and continuous scrutiny of scientific work is strengthened. From the investigator's standpoint, the care of human subjects could come to be seen as a concern secondary to the efficient and careful execution of the scientific mission, especially when society has identified others with the specific job of subject protection. The clinical researcher might then feel justified in taking what Josiah Royce called a "moral holiday," letting those charged with the care of human subjects do so and feeling quite justified in focusing only on the science.

In this way strong protectionism might inadvertently result in undermining physician investigators' sense of personal moral responsibility in the conduct of human experiments. For all the limitations of that virtue in the protection of human subjects, it is surely not one that we would want medical scientists to be without. No less an authority than the Nuremberg Code tells us so. But in spite of the stirring appeals it might still inspire, the code was a product of a long history of weak protectionism, and we shall not see that time again.

8

Convenient and Captive Populations

Clinical research is a complex, expensive, and valued social activity. One of the conditions that makes it possible is a subject population that is convenient, both in terms of availability for recruitment and for monitoring through the course of a study. Examples of such populations are prisoners, institutionalized persons, military personnel, and persons in "status relationships" (those of lesser power) such as students and research staff.[1]

Some of these populations, such as students, are convenient in the sense that they are readily available. Others are not only readily available but also captive, that is, constrained in their movements and choices by virtue of explicit conditions formally imposed on them by societal decision. The paradigm case of a captive popula-

---

1. Another sort of readily available, captive population is exemplified by the African American men who were subject to the so-called Tuskegee Syphilis Study, better named the U.S. Public Health Service Syphilis Study. These men were available and convenient by virtue of their social status. Another example is the Navajo uranium miners and millers who were observed for the carcinogenic results of their occupation for years, also by the U.S. Public Health Service. Observational studies arising from conditions that have not been created by investigators but arise in nature are also called "experiments of opportunity." See also Advisory Committee on Human Radiation Experiments (1996).

tion, of course, is those who are imprisoned. Other populations, including students, institutionalized persons, and military personnel, seem to occupy a middle ground between short-term hospitalized patients and long-term prisoners. Among the ways that these populations differ from others are their degree of availability, the greater likelihood that those who are captive can be coerced or manipulated into participation by virtue of their dependent status, and that captive populations are more likely than others to be readily available for research activities for extended periods, enhancing their attractiveness to the research enterprise.

The growing sensitivity to the use of such populations in research cannot be understood without an appreciation of the historical background. The history of research on these subject populations is important because it provides the rationale for classifying them as "vulnerable." Therefore, this chapter first reviews the historic roles of prisoners, institutionalized children and adults, military personnel, and students and staff in research activities. The discussion of each particular subject population also includes an account of the way the regulatory system has evolved to take account of historic abuses.

Because these groups are not convenient or captive—or even vulnerable—in the same ways, crafting a just, efficacious, and reasonable public policy in the use of these populations in biomedical and behavioral research is not easy. For instance, a rough notion of justice may find it acceptable to impose greater burdens on prisoners because of their debt to society. Similarly, it might be argued that those who are institutionalized may need to be used to serve some important research goal, especially if no other population so readily presents itself for study. Nevertheless, historically, these attitudes have sometimes had baleful consequences. Moreover, our intuitions about justice in research may yield inconsistent results. For example, turning soldiers into "guinea pigs" may either be offensive to patriotic sensibilities or seem reasonable in light of soldierly duties, while students and laboratory workers could be viewed either as too easily coerced into research or as the most appropriate candidates due to their ability to understand an experiment's purposes.

All these views have been represented in the history of medical research with these populations, indicating how important it has been to craft a coherent and historically informed conception of justice in research, forged to fit the special nature of convenient and captive populations. One element that crops up repeatedly in the research context is that human subjects are often used in research that is not intended to benefit them but other individuals. Likewise, a population may be used in studies that develop treatments intended mainly, or even exclusively, to benefit other groups. Any reasonably well-formed conception of justice in research will need to reckon with these special circumstances.

Discussions such as this tend to focus on ethical abuses or areas of potential moral concern. It should be remembered, however, that much human-subject research has contributed greatly to human well-being and has been conducted according to sound ethical standards. Such standards include efforts to prevent the burdens of research from falling unfairly on any particular person or group. This chapter will show how attitudes toward certain populations from which research subjects may be drawn have changed and indicate some of the issues that remain to be resolved.

JUSTICE ACROSS TIME

PRISONERS

There is none more fully captive than the long-term prisoner. Among the apocrypha of medical history are tales of the use of living criminals as subjects in various medical studies in the ancient world, including poison experiments and vivisection. In the eighteenth century, European physicians exposed prisoners to venereal disease, cancers, typhoid, and scarlet fever. An influential study of pellagra in 1914 used Mississippi convicts and presaged greater use of this population (Ethridge, 1972). During World War II in the United States, many prisoners agreed to participate in studies of conditions such as malaria and sexually transmitted diseases, partly as an expression of patriotism and partly in response to other motivations such as opportunities for payment and early parole.

After the war, a trial of those accused of conducting horrific experiments on concentration camp inmates was held in Nuremberg, West Germany. The defense attorneys in the trial pointed to cases of prison research in the United States and elsewhere as part of their justification for their clients' conduct. Among the many instances cited by the Nazis' lawyers were the pellagra and malaria studies as well as that of an American team of researchers who received permission from the governor of the Philippines to use condemned criminals and other convicts in typhus and beriberi experiments (*U.S. v. Karl Brandt et al,* 1949).

Although the Nuremberg judges sentenced some of the defendants to death and others to lengthy jail sentences for experiments on concentration camp prisoners, there was little apparent effect on the conduct of research involving American prisoners. During the Second World War American prisoners were known as, and considered to be, "volunteers," whereas the Jewish and other victims of Nazi experiments were seen as forced participants. In fact, at the same time that Illinois physician Andrew Ivy (as the AMA's representative at the trial) was authoring portions of what would become the Nuremberg Code, he also chaired a committee appointed by the governor of Illinois to review the ethics of prison research. The committee argued for constraints on the use of prisoners in research but implicitly endorsed the continued use of this population. Reporting only a few months after the Nazi doctors' trial, Ivy's committee effectively forestalled the direct application of the results of the trials to American prison research (Harkness, 1996). Several years later an early draft of the Declaration of Helsinki that would have explicitly prohibited prison research was revised at the insistence of the United States (National Commission for the Protection of Human Subjects to Biomedical and Behavioral Research, 1976).

Over the next decade several drug manufacturers made substantial investments in prison research and in some cases even erected buildings with state-of-the-art laboratory facilities at penitentiaries. By 1960 as many as 20,000 federal prisoners were participants in medical experiments (Fox, 1967). In 1973 the Pharmaceutical Manufacturers Association estimated that about 70 percent of Phase I drug tests were carried out on prisoners, or about 3,600 individuals ("Prison Research," 1973). American prisoners and prison-based facilities were also being used to test drugs for researchers abroad.

Some prison experiments were sponsored by the federal government. One involved the irradiation of the testicles of 131 prisoners in state penitentiaries in Oregon and Washington State between 1963 and 1973 and was funded by the Atomic Energy Commission. There were clear rules in place within the AEC that should have applied to these studies, including a requirement for written consent from subjects; however, in 1995 the President's Advisory Committee on Human Radiation Experiments found that these rules were not fully observed in the testicular irradiation research. Among other things, ACHRE was critical of the failure to use the word *cancer* in listing possible risks, especially with these healthy "volunteer" subjects (1996).

Among the attractions to research for prisoners were far higher pay than was afforded by other prison jobs, the possibility of a more favorable parole status, a break in the boredom of incarceration, and often better food and living conditions. A 1974 editorial in the *Journal of Legal Medicine* argued that as long as the prisoners are free to enter and leave a research program at any time, and if they understand the hazards of participation, they should be free to make this choice. The writer suggested that it would be "immoral in itself to deny them this opportunity," and "an abridgment of whatever civil and constitutional rights they may possess." So it was argued that their very rehabilitation could turn on this decision. "There is no doubt," the editorial concluded, "that biomedical research is an absolute necessity if society is to survive." Implicit in this conclusion was that prisoners are a critically important subject pool in the advancement of science (Trout, 1974).

In the mid-1970s the use of prison inmates in medical research in the United States began to decline sharply and was finally reduced almost to the point of extinction. One reason for the change in practice was a recommendation by the National Commission for the Protection of Human Subjects to Biomedical and Behavioral Research in 1976 that a moratorium be declared on prisoner experiments pending the adoption of some standards. The National Commission's recommendation followed the revelation of the Tuskegee Syphilis Study as well as a bloody prison riot at the Attica State Penitentiary in September 1971. The Attica disturbances met with a fierce response by New York State Police that left dozens of African American prisoners dead and exposed the awful living conditions to which the prisoners had been subjected. The combination of Tuskegee and Attica cast a novel and unflattering light on the coercive nature of prison life and, to many, on the coercive nature of using prisoners in research (Harkness, 1996). The National Commission's moratorium proposal met with harsh criticism from virtually every affected party: physicians, advocates, and prisoners themselves. One distinguished commentator, Louis Lasagna, charged that the National Commission's recommendations "illustrate beautifully how well-intentioned desires to protect prisoners can lead otherwise intelligent people to destroy properly performed research that scrupulously involves informed consent and full explanation and avoids coercion to the satisfaction of all but the most tunnel-visioned doctrinaire" (1977). The Department of Health, Education, and Welfare (DHEW, a predecessor to the Department of Health and Human Services) instead promulgated regulations that effectively prohibited nearly all prison research.

The premise that prison research is acceptable if prisoners are free to decline to participate is, admittedly, question-begging, and the proposition that society's survival depends on biomedical research is, if not hyperbolic, in need of defense. Yet there may be validity in the claim that research participation can forge a sense of connection to society among those who otherwise have little opportunity to feel part of any community beyond the institution. As the National Commission heard from one inmate, "It makes a prisoner feel good to volunteer. It makes him feel like he's doing something productive." But, the National Commission also heard that the primary reason for volunteering was financial, because opportunities in prison to earn money for oneself or loved ones on the outside are few (Cohn, 1976).

During the early 1990s prison research was allowable under federal regulations for only four highly restricted kinds of research: minimal risk research on incarceration and criminal behavior, studies of prisons as institutions or prisoners as incarcerated persons, research on conditions that particularly affect prisoners as a class, and studies of therapies likely to benefit the prisoner (45 C.F.R. 46, subpart C, 1993). Under the last two conditions, prison studies have been conducted on HIV/AIDS and on multiple drug-resistant tuberculosis, a disease that can occur in prisons due to the combination of the density of living conditions and a high prevalence of HIV (Potler et al., 1994).

There has therefore been a shift from well-established use of prisoners for research purposes to a protectionist regulatory framework. To find a proposed research project ethically sound, this protectionist philosophy requires a narrow construal of potential benefits to prisoners as a group or as individuals. There is considerable irony about the formation of the current public policy concerning prison research. In the most thorough scholarly analysis of the policy shift that took place in the late 1970s on the use of prisoners as subjects, historian Jon Harkness (1996) concludes that there was no contemporary social consensus on the matter. Instead, Harkness contends, retrospective consensus formed in opposition to prison research only after it had been banned by the DHEW for administrative reasons.

In this case, a widespread moral intuition seems to have come about without benefit of information about the facts of the practice in question. For example, an intuition about prison research that it invites exploitation of inmates may also lead one to believe that the most vulnerable groups in our society would be most likely to be exploited in prison research. But it is well documented that for most of the post–World War II period, African American prisoners were if anything underrepresented as prison research subjects. The reason: participation in medical experiments was considered to be a privilege that would be afforded mainly to white convicts. This situation only began to change with the success of the civil rights movement (Harkness, 1996). Similarly, by the 1960s untoward inducements for prisoner participation, such as time toward parole and high reimbursement rates, were being significantly curtailed.[2] All this suggests that, if the potential for

2. Robert J. Levine, personal communication, April 30, 1997.

coercion is taken to be the main problem of prisoners' research participation, it may not have formed a credible basis for the ultimate strict curtailment of their inclusion.

However, such a line of analysis presupposes that coercion is the only ethical problem with prison research. According to the ethical principles articulated by the National Commission for the Protection of Human Subjects in Biomedical and Behavioral Research (1974-78), the so-called Belmont principles, prison research would create ethical difficulties *even if conducted in a manner consistent with respect for persons and beneficence,* because it singles out a specific population for research participation that will then be disproportionate to that of other groups. Thus, even if the problem of coercion was resolved to our complete satisfaction, and even if we knew that participation advances the rehabilitation process, there would still be a fatal flaw. Because prisoners have in fact played a disproportionate role in research whenever and wherever such research has been permitted, their use would normally be unethical no matter how ethically satisfactory the research was in other respects.

INSTITUTIONALIZED PERSONS

The adjective "institutionalized" is used to indicate those who are chronically dependent on professional care, as compared with those for whom dependence is relatively brief and episodic, as in the case of most hospitalized patients. Persons in this category who are of particular concern to an examination of justice in research are those institutionalized persons who are cognitively impaired or mentally ill. The history of the use of these populations is considerable. For example, during the Second World War the federal Committee on Medical Research (of the White House's Office of Scientific Research and Development) approved the use of asylum patients in Mississippi in studies of influenza (Rothman, 1991).

In 1967, one year after Harvard anesthesiology professor Henry Beecher published his landmark paper identifying several instances of unethical research, British physician H. M. Pappworth described a number of ethically suspect medical experiments, among them a study of blood flow in the brains of 105 elderly demented patients. The research involved the insertion of two long needles into each jugular vein and a third in the femoral artery of the groin, and the subsequent inhaling of radioactive gas. As was true for the experiments described in the Beecher article, this study and several similar ones were published in major scientific periodicals, including the *British Medical Journal* and the *Journal of Clinical Investigation,* suggesting that research with cognitively impaired persons was both common and accepted (Pappworth, 1967).

More recently, controversy has surrounded the use of schizophrenic patients in "drug free" research, also referred to as "washout studies," in which patients are taken off psychoactive medications so that a baseline of behavior can be established and new drugs introduced to assess their effects. Public attention was called to this practice by the suicide of a patient who had been a subject in such a study at the University of California at Los Angeles two years before. In their investigation of the UCLA study, the federal Office for Protection from Research Risks (OPRR) found nothing unethical in the conduct of the research but was critical of the consent form's failure to indicate clearly that a patient's schizophrenic symptoms may recur (Shamoo and Keay, 1996).

Although federal regulations were codified for prisoners in 1981, there are no federal regulations concerning the use of adults with diminished decision-making capacity, in spite of the National Commission's recommendations concerning this population. As a result, conditions for the ethical participation of incapacitated adults in research are unsettled, not only for those whose source of incapacity is mental illness but also for those who become incapacitated secondary to another medical condition.

However, public interest in revisiting the regulation of research with those who are "decisionally impaired" seems to be building (R. Levine, 1997; Bonnie, 1997). One element of this trend is the growing promise of interventions in Alzheimer's disease and associated dementias. These persons have varying degrees of capacity, and it is argued that their mental status should be no reason for excluding them from their best therapeutic hope, namely, the interventions available through research. At least two sets of ethics guidelines have been suggested for research with this population

(High et al., 1994; Keyserlingk, 1995). While some advocate regulation that would enable research to proceed with greater confidence, others emphasize the risks associated with some research strategies, such as "drug holidays," in which psychoactive medications are withdrawn so that the patient returns to a baseline level of functioning (*T.D. v. State Office of Metal Health,* 1996). To some degree, this difference of opinion about the need for protection for the decisionally impaired may stem from the specific study population, with greater support of research coming from those interested in conditions such as Alzheimer's disease, as compared with psychiatric diseases such as schizophrenia.

Institutionalized children include mentally infirm minors as well as those who are simply indigent. Whatever the reason for their institutionalization, these children are captive in a double sense, for not only are they dependent on the care of others in an artificial setting, but they are also legally and often practically incapable of making meaningful decisions on their own behalf. Therefore, decisions to permit their participation in medical research are generally out of their hands and are the province of a parent or legal guardian. Frequently in the history of research with institutionalized children, the state has been the decision maker.

In 1759 Francis Home, a Scottish physician, attempted to protect twelve children from measles by inoculating them with blood taken from a measles patient, having promised a payment to their parents (Still, 1965). During the next hundred years several other similar efforts to prevent measles were made with children, including residents of a Chicago orphan asylum (Cassidy, 1984). At the end of the eighteenth century, Edward Jenner tested his smallpox vaccine on his one-year-old son. Institutionalized children were then used to test Jenner's vaccine when Thomas C. James inoculated forty-eight children in the Philadelphia almshouse in 1802 (Radbill, 1979). The growing interest in diseases of childhood throughout the nineteenth century found ready research and training sites in the increasing number of schools, orphanages, reformatories, and foundling homes. Studies on institutionalized children were undertaken for pellagra, sexually transmissible diseases, scarlet fever, diphtheria, tuberculosis, chickenpox, mumps, and whooping cough (Lederer and Grodin, 1994).

By the turn of the century new technologies were being developed and applied to the study of the basic physiology of children, among them x-rays for the investigation of internal organs and stomach tubes for research on the mechanisms of digestion. Changing attitudes toward children and childhood during the first decades of the twentieth century soon heightened public suspicion of research practices, including the use of those who were institutionalized. In 1914, for instance, a Rockefeller Institute scientist used orphans in trials of a new test for syphilis. The New York Society for the Prevention of Cruelty to Children filed a complaint with the District Attorney. Although it was admitted that the physicians involved lacked authority to give consent, the charges were dropped. Calls to outlaw "vivisectionism" in children also resulted in proposed laws in the U.S. Senate and several state legislatures, none of which were passed.

Nevertheless, during World War II the federal Committee on Medical Research, an arm of the Executive Office of the President, funded a number of studies in which children were subjects. In 1943, at an Ohio orphanage that was the site of research on dysentery, injections of killed bacteria caused serious side effects in some of the children (Lederer and Grodin, 1994).

The most infamous recent study, involving institutionalized children at Willowbrook State School on Staten Island, New York, continues to excite controversy about its ethical standing. From the late 1950s to the early 1970s Dr. Saul Krugman and his team of infectious disease specialists from New York University conducted hepatitis research at Willowbrook. Most Willowbrook residents were severely mentally retarded and developed hepatitis through exposure to the body fluids of other children at the school. In order to study the natural history of the virus and in the hopes of developing a prophylaxis, Krugman and his colleagues systematically infected some newly admitted children with the virus. Parental consent was obtained, but Krugman was later criticized because those who agreed to have their children serve as research subjects were granted more rapid admission for their profoundly disabled children. Though scholarly opinion about the ethics of Willowbrook remains unsettled, and Krugman himself issued a spirited defense of his methods (Krugman 1986), it was one of the incidents that aroused public concern and advanced moves for greater federal regulation in the 1970s.

Although the details did not emerge until the mid-1990s, in the late 1940s and early 1950s the Atomic Energy Commission sponsored secret cold war nutritional studies using institutionalized adolescents in cooperation with the makers of Quaker Oats cereal. The residents of the Fernald School in Waltham, Massachusetts, were adolescents, but not as seriously disabled as those at Willowbrook. The work was performed by researchers from the Massachusetts Institute of Technology. Trace elements of radiation were introduced into the meals of male residents. Parents who gave their permission were told that their children would be in a "science club" that would include special meals, extra milk, and field trips, but not that radiation was involved.

The Fernald studies were subjected to official investigations many years later at both the state and federal levels. The Massachusetts Task Force on Human Subject Research concluded in 1994 that the researchers did not provide the students and their families with information critical to making an informed decision to participate in the studies. In 1995 the ACHRE concluded that the Fernald research and a similar project at the Wrentham School "unfairly burdened children who were already disadvantaged, children whose interests were less well protected than those children living with their parents, or children who were socially privileged."

Current rules governing federally funded pediatric research grew out of concerns stimulated by revelation of the Willowbrook experiment and other cases. In the end, the National Commission's recommendations became the template for the rules that are now in place.[3]

3. The current regulations are relatively detailed, though parents, investigators, and institutional review boards are still given wide latitude to approve studies. Using a "sliding scale" approach, restrictions vary according to the ratio of risk and benefit. Most difficult to perform with children is research involving significant risks that do not present the prospect of directly benefiting the subject. Certain kinds of research, such as anonymous educational test results, are exempt from the federal rules. Perhaps the most problematic concept in the pediatric regulations is that of minimal risk, upon which the permissibility of much research turns. In the federal rules, risk is said to be minimal when it does not exceed that encountered in daily life or in a regular physical or psychological examination, a standard that may not be very protective in light of the many hazards of ordinary childhood. Another feature of the current regulations that blunts their force is the absence of a requirement that investigators show that the work can only be done with children, unlike the prisoner requirements. See also Leonard H. Glantz, "The Law of Experimentation with Children," in Grodin and Glantz, 1994, pp. 123–25.

MILITARY PERSONNEL

Military personnel are convenient subjects in the sense that they are typically healthy, "normal" persons who can be followed for data collection for a number of years. However, their disciplined environment raises questions about the extent to which any consent they give can be considered truly voluntary. Thus, they may be at risk for disproportionate representation in research, especially in studies relating to national security. Yet military officials have long considered voluntariness an important condition for participation in research by military personnel, as evidenced by the use of the term "volunteer" or "informed volunteer" from at least the 1940s (ACHRE, 1996). The precise significance to be given the term under the circumstances is, of course, a separate but vitally important matter.

The American record in the use of military personnel in research has been mixed—a history of pioneering policies inconsistently applied. Around 1900, U.S. Army scientist Walter Reed obtained consent and asked potential subjects to sign a written contract for his yellow fever experiment in Cuba. The contract specified some of the risks and offered nonmilitary personnel monetary compensation for participating; soldiers reportedly declined the compensation. The $200 in gold that Reed offered the Spanish workers who participated in the experiment was a significant amount of money at the time, perhaps enough to be considered coercive today. There was little opportunity to withdraw from the study. Reed's colleagues (but not Reed himself) on the Yellow Fever Commission also subjected themselves to the mosquito's bite that was correctly suspected as the source of the infection. One of Reed's colleagues died of the infection.

Though Reed began his dangerous experiment without his superior's approval, he felt obligated to ask his commanding officer's permission when he thought it necessary to expand the study. Since at least the 1930s it appears that approval for soldiers' and sailors' participation in medical experiments was to be obtained at the highest level of the relevant uniformed service, usually from the service's surgeon general and often from the service secretary as well. The assignment of military personnel to research is, after all, a deployment decision that should theoretically be made by the responsible officer in the chain of command.

There are also significant potential risks to the armed forces if an experiment goes awry, especially in terms of public opinion and legal liability, another reason for proper authorization of human research. During the Second World War, the Committee on Medical Research declared that uniformed personnel were not to be used as "guinea pigs" in the war-related research it funded. Throughout this period there was significant concern that the public would not be sympathetic if their heroes were to be used in this manner. Nonetheless, during the war naval personnel were forced to remain in mustard gas experiments against their will.

By the late 1940s there was a growing view in the national security establishment that some human experiments were going to be necessary in the postwar environment, especially in reference to unconventional weapons: atomic, biological, and chemical. The effects of these weapons could not be gauged in animal studies, nor could their combat implications be assessed with other healthy subjects. Early 1950s studies of flash blindness following atomic detonations, for example, were classified by the Pentagon as medical experiments, though most other exposures to the atomic battlefield were considered to be part of necessary training (ACHRE, 1996).

The Department of Defense attempted to anticipate the problem of using military personnel in research by adopting the Nuremberg Code as its policy in 1953. Subsequently, troops deployed near the site of atomic tests were systematically observed, and they sometimes filed self-reports of panic reactions near the blast site. "Release" forms were even filled out in at least some cases by troops who had "volunteered" to operate closer to ground zero than others, thus exposing themselves to a higher level of radioactivity. Yet in other studies involving military personnel and radiation there was no documentation of volunteer status except the statements of superior officers (ACHRE, 1996). In still other cases, such as the air force's mushroom cloud penetration experiments that measured the amount of fission released by an atomic blast and its effects on crew members, there is strong evidence that at least some air force personnel were eager to experience the challenge and adventure associated with the project, while others viewed the job as part of their routine.

The military context presents a unique puzzle about distinguishing training, which does not typically fall under the constraints of medical ethics, from medical research, which does. For instance, the vast majority of the "atomic soldiers" deployed for exercises at the training facility at Camp Desert Rock in Nevada from 1951 to 1962 were kept at what was thought to be a safe distance from the atomic blast site. Though any acute ill effects might have been noted, the primary goal of the activity was to learn about human factors such as panic reactions on the atomic battlefield. Although the tension between national security needs and ethical considerations was rarely a topic of public discussion during the cold war, it played an important role in shaping the defense establishment's ambivalent posture toward human subjects issues (ACHRE, 1996).

The implementation of the Nuremberg Code–based policy appears to have been sporadic at best, perhaps partly because there was confusion about its scope and application. The Army Inspector General found in 1975 that the army had failed to comply with its own rules for the use of soldiers in research with psychoactive drugs when thousands of men at Fort Detrick, Maryland, were used in LSD experiments in the 1950s (Downey, 1975). Even in the courts, the Code has not proven to be an effective standard. When one of the men brought suit against the U.S. government for injuries he incurred due to this research, the Supreme Court ruled in favor of the government by a five-to-four majority on the grounds that the judicial branch should not undermine discipline by inquiring into military matters. Only the minority argued that the Nuremberg Code must prevail (*U.S. v. Stanley,* 1987).

Today, medical research in the armed forces has both reduced its dependence on healthy, "normal" subjects and, like other sectors of American society, has established a very low threshold of risk tolerance in the development of new armaments, equipment, and materials. In 1991 the Department of Defense regulations on the use of human subjects were brought under the same requirements as other federal agencies that sponsor studies with human subjects (*Federal Policy for the Protection of Human Subjects,* 1991). The additional regulatory obstacles to recruitment of military personnel for research are such that today this is among the most difficult populations from which to obtain subjects. Today, all research in the army's infectious disease institute at Fort Detrick, for example, is governed by several regulations, and proposals involving significant risk must be reviewed by a local institutional review board (IRB), the Human Use Review and Regulatory Affairs Division of the United States Army Medical Research and Material Command, the Human Subjects Research Review Board of the Office of the Surgeon General, and the Office of the Surgeon General itself (USAMRIID Reg. No. 70-52, 4.b). In response to the recommendations of the ACHRE, in 1997 President Clinton ordered expanded training for senior officers on the nature of human subjects research and instituted a new policy that precludes officers from involvement in the recruitment of research volunteers (US Government Human Radiation Interagency Working Group, 1997).

Other recent events illustrate the special ethical difficulties associated with regulating the use of innovative drugs with military personnel during a national emergency. In late 1990 and early 1991 during Operation Desert Shield and Desert Storm, the Defense Department was concerned about possible exposure to biological and chemical warfare agents. The department successfully sought an amendment to the FDA's informed consent regulations that would enable medical professionals to determine that it was "not feasible" to obtain the informed consent of a person receiving an investigational drug or vaccine under combat conditions. The rule was published on December 21, 1990, and upheld by the courts (Advisory Committee on Gulf War Veteran's Illnesses, 1996).

Shortly after the rule was published, the Department of Defense requested and received waivers of informed consent for two investigational products: pyriodostigmine bromide (PB) and botulinum toxoid (BT). Even though the waiver was obtained for both agents, Central Command elected on ethical grounds to give service personnel a choice about receiving BT, but not for PB, which was in common use as an approved drug for other populations and for which informed consent was not deemed necessary. The Pentagon estimates that about 8,000 troops took BT and about 250,000 received at least one dose of PB (Advisory Committee on Gulf War Veteran's Illnesses, 1996).

Months after the war, some veterans began complaining about numerous symptoms that when grouped together are termed "Gulf War Syndrome." The vaccination program was shrouded in secrecy when it took place to deny information to the enemy about the Allies' defensive measures, but as the story emerged, the agents, especially PB, were theorized by some as a factor in the veterans' medical problems. A federal advisory committee was appointed to investigate the health problems of Gulf War veterans, including an analysis of the waiver process (Advisory Committee on Gulf War Veteran's Illnesses, 1996b).

However skeptical one might be about such claims of voluntariness against an admitted record of pressuring uniformed personnel to "volunteer," matters surely become far more complicated in the case of potentially prophylactic agents used under combat conditions. In this case it can be argued that access to compounds that have not yet been approved for use under ordinary circumstances may be ethical. The lack of approval could be due to technical or bureaucratic factors, and there may be sound scientific evidence that the agent can be of significant potential benefit to troops in battle (C. Levine, 1989).

Underlying much of the criticism of the Pentagon's conduct in the use of unapproved drugs is a suspicion that it was a deliberate effort to circumvent research requirements in order to assess the agents' efficacy under combat conditions. There is no evidence that this is the case. Indeed, one shortcoming of the Defense Department's handling of this episode is precisely the fact that no system was in place to document the response of service personnel to the medications, including a failure to establish appropriate baseline measures of subjects' metabolism (Advisory Committee on Gulf War Veteran's Illnesses, 1996—Final Report). The use of these compounds "in theater" could theoretically have been justified on scientific as well as beneficent grounds if the operation had been treated as a research study according to established methodological standards.

Had a systematic research dimension been part of the agents' use in Desert Storm, there then would have been an opportunity to assess the fairness of conducting research with military personnel. The assessment would have turned on the manner in which the study was conducted, for while soldiers facing combat conditions may be required to accept all medical interventions that hold the prospect of ensuring their availability for service, the innovative use of these drugs may not entail a requirement to accept them. But if the decision to use the agents could have been left to the troops themselves, with appropriate information at their disposal about known risks and benefits, then their participation would have been acceptable. Apparently this information was not made available in Desert Storm, in spite of an agreement between the Defense Department and the FDA that it would be provided (US House of Representatives, 1997).

STUDENTS

Students are captive in a different sense from any of the groups mentioned thus far. They exemplify persons who are not literally captive, and may even be among our most privileged citizens, but are in a social context characterized by power relations. In particular, their differential role is characterized by inherently lesser power than the other member of the relationship, in this instance a teacher. Students are by no means unique in this sense; other relationships that are characterized by power differentials are employers and employees, and supervisors and laboratory workers. In general, whatever recruitment policies are established for students in research will tend to apply to those who are similarly vulnerable by virtue of other power relationships.

The potentially coercive nature of being a student may arise from a course requirement that they serve as a study subject. Or they may respond to campus or local advertisements offering cash in exchange for volunteering for research. Since students are often unemployed or underemployed, even small monetary inducements can be important. Perhaps because the kind of research to which students are usually subjected is behavioral and presents minimal physical risk (though arguably some psychological risk) and there has been no great scandal about participation in studies as a course requirement, this population has received the least attention among those that may be said to be in a coercive environment.

Some of the studies to which students are most likely to be exposed, especially undergraduates recruited for social science experiments, fall into the category known as "deception research." Social psychological studies involving deception increased greatly through the 1950s and 1960s. Few expressed concern about the ethical implications of deceit or the potential psychological damage to the subject until the mid-1960s, following Stanley Milgram's studies of obedience (Milgram, 1974). Milgram's basic design called for two people to be told they were participating in a memory experiment, but one of the two was a "confederate," a member of the research team. The naïve actual subject was instructed to shock the other "subject" (the confederate) if he or she failed to give the correct answer to word-pair questions. Most of the actual subjects gave the confederates "shocks" they were led to believe were dangerous because the experimenter told them to follow through on the punishment for making a mistake (Milgram, 1974).

In the years following publication, the scientific importance of Milgram's studies vied for attention with the ethical issues they raised. Many critics expressed concern about the emotional well-being of the subjects once they realized both that they had been deceived and that they were evidently capable of inflicting harm on innocent people merely because they were instructed to do so by an authority figure, a scientist. There was no informed consent about this aspect of the research, and it is hard to see how there could be without confounding the study.

Another celebrated deception research case heightened the debate shortly after Milgram's original publication, when in the late 1960s sociologist Laud Humphreys conducted research on the social status of those engaging in anonymous homosexual encounters in public restrooms. His data-gathering techniques included secretly recording car license numbers and later presenting himself in the subjects' homes posing as a health services researcher and asking questions about their personal lives. Humphreys succeeded in undermining numerous false stereotypes about gay men, but his approach caused an uproar that reached beyond his department and university to national newspapers (Humphreys, 1970).

Obviously these famous cases are fairly extreme examples of deception studies, and they do not necessarily involve students, whose research participation is likely to occur under more benign circumstances. The American Psychological Association's code of ethics continues to permit deception in research and does not address the disproportionate use of "captive" populations such as those who may be required to serve as research subjects as part of satisfying a course requirement (APA, 1982).

Of the students who may be asked to participate as subjects in research, a smaller number is engaged in advanced biological or medical studies. In one sense they are close to ideal candidates because of their potential intellectual identification with the research; the only superior subjects in this sense are the principal investigators themselves (Jonas, 1970). The creation of special obstacles to the enrollment of these students, who are generally regarded as the "best and the brightest" by their faculties and far less likely to be exploited than other societal groups, may be viewed as institutional paternalism (Christakis, 1985). Nevertheless, there is evidence that medical students do not believe their professors' consent processes are adequate (Kopelman, 1993).

Finally, there is again the issue of financial compensation. In order to avoid appearing coercive, remuneration for study participation should take into account the financial position of the population from which subjects are to be recruited. Many students live on loans that present them with a significant burden for many years. In the first instance, compensation may take into account expenses associated with study participation, such as travel. Additional amounts should be calculated based on a reasonable assessment of the value of the time invested by members of that population. Thus, for example, one hundred dollars an hour for an individual who could not otherwise earn a fraction of that amount would seem to be coercive.

FUTURE TRENDS

Because they are captive in very different ways, determining justice in research with these subject populations must be assessed quite differently. We have seen that the ready availability of institutionalized subjects like prisoners makes them prime research candidates, a circumstance that applies even more powerfully to those in medical institutions, for they have already been identified as in need of medical attention. The population of potential subjects in medical institutions is a complex one both because of the different ages and levels of capacity and because all the research for which they may be recruited will involve manipulations or procedures intended to benefit them in spite of the fact that they are ill.

Surely the subpopulation in this large and diverse group that is a likely candidate for new or expanded regulatory protections in the future is the mentally infirm, understood as those with chronic rather than acute cognitive deficits, such as Alzheimer's disease or schizophrenia; or, in the case of minors, deficits related to factors other than immaturity alone, such as mental retardation. A recent legal case at the state level, nonbeneficial research on patients in New York State psychiatric hospitals, invalidated regulations that permitted greater than minimal risk (*T.D. v. State Office of Mental Health,* 1996). This case, and continuing uncertainty among investigators over consent procedures for important research with the mentally infirm, has caught the attention of the National Bioethics Advisory Commission (NBAC), which is likely to recommend some regulatory reform. Considering the absence of rules targeted to this population, it seems likely that almost any explicit regulations will create more rather than fewer obstacles to their use. Thus, one can expect that locales in which much psychiatric research was done with patients in the past will be doing fewer studies, or using fewer patients, in the future.

Since the Gulf War, a primary public policy concern has revolved around waivers of informed consent provisions involving unapproved drugs for military personnel under combat conditions. The suitability of such waivers may be loosely characterized as a matter of justice in research, but only if the program for which a waiver is sought is intended mainly to yield information that can be used in later conflicts. Considering that the primary goal of the waiver is not research (and indeed medical data-gathering was not part of the Pentagon's mission in Desert Storm), the problem here does not seem to be one of discrimination against soldiers as disproportionately recruited to be experimental subjects. Rather, the dilemma stems from a wish to provide the troops with whatever medical benefit might theoretically be available without unacceptable risk.

More pertinent to the topic of justice in research for the military in the future is whether and under what conditions men and women in the armed forces may be utilized in new research activities during peacetime. In general, for both political and moral reasons there has been a reluctance to use military personnel in research when others are available. This reluctance has been compromised when some new threat seemed imminent and other appropriate subjects were not available. Therefore, a source of tension in the future about the acceptance of using military personnel in research could be a suspected new and deadly weapons system in the possession of a foreign power or terrorist group, combined with regulatory restrictions on the use of other healthy subjects.

Considering how much use is made of young people like students in medical and behavioral research, a few isolated tragedies can excite considerable public alarm. Some further restrictions on the use of students in research seem likely, at least at local levels, perhaps by prohibiting their recruitment by their current instructors. In 1996 a 19-year-old University of Rochester undergraduate died after participating in a study involving a bronchoscopy; the young woman succumbed two days following a reaction to a local anesthetic. She was to be paid $150 as a normal volunteer. Although harm to student volunteers is extremely rare and mortality is a virtually unheard-of event, this case has excited understandable concern in New York. The state health commissioner appointed a panel to review the use of normal subjects and recommend improvements in the IRB system ("New York seeks to tighten rules," 1996).

CONCLUSIONS

Generalized discussions about justice are sorely limited concerning specific groups. In crafting a just public policy for the use of human subjects, especially those who may be considered convenient or captive, the historical and practical factors that could enter into judgments about justice will vary depending on what population is being considered. The respective situations of prisoners, institutionalized persons, military personnel, and students are quite different and require analyses tailored to each of them. Underlying all of these cases are complex issues of social status and power as well as medical ethics.

As experience in modern research with human subjects has accumulated, a "protectionist" attitude toward the participation of these groups has emerged. Prisoners are no longer a rich source of subjects, and specific federal regulations greatly restrict their involvement in studies. Institutionalized persons have long been considered to generate specific ethical issues in research, a trend that has lately accelerated. Research with military personnel, always a sensitive problem for defense officials, must navigate numerous obstacles for approval by command authorities. Participation in research by students, employees, and others in differential power positions is a simmering issue that may well be the next frontier for protectionist approaches.

Historical experience has been accompanied by an evolution in the sense of justice in research, one that has tended to qualify crude utilitarian attitudes toward the use of human subjects. The notion that long-term prisoners owe a special debt to society that may be expressed in research participation, for example, is an implication of a once-popular notion of justice that has resonance only to the degree that it is abstracted from actual abuses associated with imprisonment, including the familiar problem of voluntariness. Similarly, the view that prisoners or other institutionalized persons may have to be used in risky studies addressing important public health problems must be tempered by the condition (already in current regulations) that they must themselves be likely to benefit from such research, either as individuals or, at the very least, as members of the affected group.

Once a more refined conception of justice in research becomes available, it may have implications for groups it was not even intended to address. The notion that military service does not include duties to be in research that is not intended to improve combat readiness is one that the armed forces were already coming to accept by the mid-1970s, but the Tuskegee Syphilis Study scandal and the work of the National Commission surely helped to reinforce an awareness of research ethics in the military, as it did in all other areas. Under the auspices of a modern conception of justice in research, the proposition that the role of student or employee does not generate an obligation to serve in an experiment is now becoming more obvious.

A protectionist stance toward special populations does not rule out the possibility that strong arguments for research participation can be mounted. Surely there are circumstances in which justice may permit, or even require, access to research for populations that have historically been abused by some researchers. One of these circumstances is the prevalence of a disease that poses a particular threat to members of that population and that cannot be studied as effectively with other subjects. Protected status implies institutional and public scrutiny of proposed research participation, not a priori exclusion. With this understanding, and in light of the historical factors that have made these groups' participation in medical research a matter of special concern, protectionism continues to be a morally sound presumption.

9

Regulation of Research in the
Decisionally Impaired

The term "decisionally impaired" poses a recurring definitional problem. All of us are going to be decisionally impaired at one time or another. The causes could be many: immaturity, disease, the secondary effects of medication, or disorienting life events, among others. This chapter will focus on the kind of decisional impairment that is chronic rather than acute, and pathological rather than associated with "normal" youth or aging. I readily grant that there can be exceptions to this generalization, but it may help us avoid entering into related but distinct issues and populations, such as decision making for those in the emergency setting (usually an acute and not chronic decisional deficit), or for those who are very young (usually normal and not pathological).

With this rough delimiting framework as a guide, I will attempt to develop an outline of the history and ethics of research regulation with this heterogeneous population. In developing this outline, I encountered an unhappy fact about the scholarship in this area that the present paper is intended to help ameliorate.

There is, so far as I can tell, no authoritative history of the use in biomedical and behavioral research of persons who are decisionally impaired, nor is this population commonly identified in the historical literature as distinctly at risk for involvement in a study. This scholarly neglect now shows signs of abating, as does the neglect of this population in the policy arena.

PERSONAL ORIENTATION TO HUMAN SUBJECTS RESEARCH

While readers with an interest in this topic may be aware of my work on the history and ethics of research with human subjects (J. D. Moreno, 1997; Faden et al., 1996; Moreno and Lederer, 1996; Moreno, 1996b, c), they may not realize that my interest in research with those who are decisionally impaired began when I was about ten years old. My father, J. L. Moreno, was a distinguished psychiatrist who pioneered the fields of group psychotherapy, psychodrama, sociometry, and role playing (Marineau, 1989). I grew up on the banks of the Hudson River in Beacon, New York, on a 20-acre tract that included a small psychiatric hospital that my father modeled on the European sanitariums he knew as a medical student in Vienna. My home was about 80 yards from the hospital. Although my parents tried to keep me an appropriate distance from the patients, my earliest friends included persons with schizophrenia, manic-depression, drug addictions, senile dementia, and other neurological disorders.

One day in 1962 a busload of young people arrived on the grounds. Patients of my father's colleague in Manhattan, they were to participate in a special therapy weekend at the Moreno Sanitarium. I remember organizing a softball game after they got settled, and one young man remarked that the place seemed pretty good. "Yeah," another fellow replied, "but once they start giving you the stuff, it'll be just like anywhere else." The remark stuck with me, perhaps because I was a little hurt by it, but also I wondered what "the stuff" was, especially that weekend. My father did not work much with drugs; he was too old-fashioned to accept wholeheartedly the pharmacologic revolution in psychiatry.

Later I learned that "the stuff" in question that weekend was a hallucinogen that later became a symbol of an era but was unknown to most people at the time. It was lysergic acid diethyla-mide, LSD-25. The goal was to examine its effect as an adjunct to group psychotherapy. Evidently, the results were disappointing. According to my mother, a well-known therapist who also worked with the patients that weekend, it was too hard to tell where the drug left off and the personality began. Neither of my parents took the drug themselves. My father's former Harvard colleague, then Hudson Valley neighbor, Timothy Leary, later proved a more willing guide to the psychedelic world to come.

That weekend on the Hudson I witnessed a gathering for thera-peutic research. I have since wondered what sort of consent pro-cess was involved when the patients were recruited for the LSD-cum-psychotherapy weekend. I do know that my father was aware of, and troubled by, these issues. His compassion for his patients, with whom he identified far more than with his professional col-leagues, contributed to his reputation as a maverick. In the mem-oirs he completed shortly before his death in 1974, he recalled his work as a second-year medical student in the clinic of Julius Wag-ner von Jauregg, an important figure in the history of psychiatric research. The year was probably 1915, and the place was Vienna, Austria, but the culture of academic medicine sounds familiar:

> There was no salary for being a research assistant at the clinic, just a tremendous opportunity to meet and to work with some of the top psychiatrists, both research and clinical, in the world, and, in my case, to have my name on publications, still an important fac-tor in a young scientist's career. I was involved in a few other re-search projects there, but the only one I remember is a study of iodine metabolism. We went to the Tyrol and injected rats full of iodine. . . . After experimenting on rats, we experimented on in-mates at the psychiatric hospital connected with the Von Jauregg clinic, Steinhoff hospital.
>
> I have always been appalled at the idea of experimenting on helpless mental patients. I remember projects—I was not involved with them—in which patients were injected with TB bacilli and another in which injections of alcohol were administered. (J. L. Moreno, 1987)

Shortly after the incidents my father recalled, in his graduation year 1917, his mentor, Wagner von Jauregg, experimented with the induction of fevers as a cure for general paresis, a condition that occurs during the tertiary phase of syphilis and can cause insanity, paralysis, and death (J. L. Moreno, 1987). He injected nine paralyzed patients with malaria, which was subsequently cured with quinine. The malaria-induced fevers were claimed to cure a large percentage of the patients. For his discovery, Wagner von Jauregg was awarded the Nobel Prize for Medicine or Physiology in 1927, and malaria therapy for general paresis has since been superseded by penicillin therapy.

Important as it was, Wagner von Jauregg's work was clouded by his questionable use of mentally ill patients as research subjects, a practice that was apparently common in Austrian psychiatry and neurology at the time. Interestingly, Wagner von Jauregg himself was an ardent campaigner for laws to protect the insane from persecution and discrimination. Physicians in that part of the world must have been well aware of problems in research ethics. In 1892 a Prussian medical school professor had given blood serum from people with syphilis to four children and three young prostitutes. Dr. Albert Neisser worked on a syphilis vaccine but failed to ask the permission of those he infected or their legal guardians. When several contracted the disease, newspapers carried banner headlines about the scandal. In 1900 the Prussian government directed that medical research must have the human subject's consent (Grodin, 1992).

RESEARCH WITH SICK PATIENTS

Historically, experiments with sick patients afflicted with the disease being studied have not been perceived as bound by the same ethical constraints as research with healthy, "normal" subjects. This longstanding perception has also been examined in another context by the federal Advisory Committee on Human Radiation Experiments, which reported to President Clinton in October 1995 on government-sponsored studies of ionizing radiation. If this reconstruction of an historical assumption is correct (an assumption of which people may not, of course, have been aware at the time), it may help to explain why certain very public experimental uses of the decisionally impaired rarely provoked a general outrage: They were assumed to fall within the then-privileged domain of doctor-patient relationships.

The only other Nobelist in psychiatry, Portuguese physician Egas Moniz, who won in 1949 for Physiology or Medicine, also engaged in experiments with sick patients (Wasson and Brieger, 1987). American physiologists had experimented with monkeys by surgically removing their prefrontal lobes. As a result, the monkeys no longer became upset when they made mistakes carrying out complex tasks they had learned; they seemed to be immune to anxiety and frustration. Moniz theorized that the same might be true for severely anxious or aggressive mental patients. The operation did seem to cure at least some of the first twenty on whom it was tried.[1] Moniz was forced to supervise the performance of more than one hundred "leucotomies" (later called lobotomies) because he was too impaired by gout in his hands to perform the procedure himself.[2] The technique was eventually banned by the Portuguese government, but others adopted it and it was widely used, especially in the United States.

Several more innovative somatic therapies were introduced into psychiatry in the 1930s. "Shock therapy" involves electrical impulses or drugs such as insulin to induce hypoglycemia, or metrazol to induce convulsions. Contemporary psychiatrists were discomfited by the rush of these new and unproven drastic interventions. As historian Gerald Grob (1994) stated, physicians asked whether they should "deploy experimental therapies on patients whose illness often impaired their mental faculties?" Finally, the pressure to find an effective treatment for the large number of chronic mental patients crowding hospitals in this era of institutionalization overwhelmed such abstract questions. In Grob's words, "If there was even a remote chance that an experimental therapy would aid them, should they be deprived of its use until more conclusive evidence was available?" In the history of research

---

1. Of the first twenty operations, seven of the patients were considered cured, eight improved, and five were unchanged.

2. Moniz dubbed the procedure a "leucotomy," from the Greek word for white, because of the white matter connecting the prefrontal lobes to other parts of the brain that were surgically removed.

ethics, this argument is a familiar, and to some degree compelling, rationale.

The iconic status of the Nobel Prize serves to highlight the complex ethical issues at the heart of the only two Nobels given in psychiatry.[3] But the centrality of these issues in our cultural history extends well beyond these examples. They are embedded in the development of modern liberal democratic society itself, and in the context of public policy toward the mentally ill. One of the signal events of the French Revolution was the freeing of the inmates of the asylum of Salpetriere by Philippe Pinel, who believed, consistent with the revolutionary philosophy, that insanity would be cured by the establishment of an new civil society (J. D. Moreno, 1981). Some trace to this incident the beginning of the moral treatment movement that dominated the care of the mentally ill for a hundred years, evolving finally into the mental hygiene movement of the early twentieth century. Alexis de Tocqueville, one of the most renowned commentators on the American scene, arrived specifically to report on the way the new country was managing its most marginal citizens in new asylums. Moral treatment institutions were carefully designed to provide "lunatics" with the social and physical orderliness that might imprint itself on their disordered brains. The moral treatment movement was a grand and well-meaning, albeit unsystematic, social experiment with the seemingly recalcitrant problem of mental illness.[4]

Other innovations in the eighteenth and nineteenth centuries more closely resembled therapeutic research because they were directed specifically toward mentally ill patients (J. D. Moreno, 1981). Some of these techniques were practiced in moral treatment institutions in spite of their apparent philosophical inconsistency. Bloodletting, purging with emetics, and shock therapy all had their day; and had controlled research methods been available, that day would probably have been shorter in every case. When the resources of the new biologically based medicine combined with randomized controlled trials, a powerful new weapon

3. I am indebted to my SUNY colleague, Dinko Podrug, M.D., for this point.
4. Similar charges have been lodged against a more recent policy response to mental illness, de-institutionalization. Like moral treatment, de-institutionalization was a large-scale social experiment that did not meet the statutory definition of research.

was theoretically available to psychiatry and neurology as to other disciplines. But until the mid-twentieth century, there remained a frustrating lack of potential drug therapies. Controlled studies of cognitively and socially oriented interventions like psychoanalysis and psychotherapy are notoriously difficult to perform with reliability because of the countless variables that affect these processes.

Finally, in the early 1950s, there was hope for the long-sought medical treatment of mental disorders. A class of tranquilizers gained notoriety for ameliorating the symptoms of schizophrenia (Brown, 1985). But here too, the human research issue casts a shadow. The neuroleptic drugs unquestionably inaugurated a new era in the treatment of the mentally ill, and by the mid-1970s the de-institutionalization policy they helped justify was well established. Unfortunately, the new "psychoactive" medications also had serious side effects with long-term use, a fact that was recognized by the 1960s. Some commentators charged that the drug company that marketed Thorazine, the first of these medications, conducted hasty clinical trials in its rush to bring the potentially lucrative new product to market. These charges followed the thalidomide tragedy that resulted in the subsequent expansion of the U.S. Food and Drug Administration's authority to include efficacy as well as toxicity in approving the sale of drugs (Federal Food, Drug and Cosmetic Act, 1997). In the case of Thorazine, like thalidomide, the problem was not conducting overly aggressive clinical research, but just the opposite (though thalidomide's teratogenicity was so statistically infrequent that only a massive, large-scale study would have uncovered it). The alleged result was the wide prescription of a psychiatric medication whose long-term effects were not well understood, and which justified a drastically altered social policy, and in effect ignited another social experiment, directed at the perennial problem of mental illness.

THE DECISIONALLY IMPAIRED AND NONTHERAPEUTIC RESEARCH

Not all instances of ethically questionable research practices involving those who are decisionally impaired are intended to benefit the subjects, nor are they intended to yield knowledge of the sources of the impairment that affect the subject population. Rather, they may have an entirely unrelated purpose, such as determining the effects of an agent on the human body, or the body's effect on the agent. In these cases the decisionally impaired subject is chosen for research because he or she is readily available, especially if the subject is institutionalized. Two prominent illustrations of this scenario occurred during the 1950s, though they were generally known only much later.

In 1952, Harold Blauer was a 42-year-old jet-setting tennis pro at Manhattan's Hudson River Club (*Barrett v. U.S.*, 1987). Sometime that summer, Blauer was divorced from his wife and became, in the fall, a patient of Bellevue Hospital. He was diagnosed with clinical depression and was admitted voluntarily to the New York State Psychiatric Institute. Blauer was not aware that the NYPI had a secret contract with the Army Chemical Corps to conduct research using a mescaline derivative.[5] In mid-January of 1953, Blauer was given a number of injections with widely varying doses, of which the last one was significantly larger than the first. Blauer went into convulsions and died hours later. The army and New York State arranged a cover-up of the actual circumstances of Blauer's death and split an $18,000 payment[6] between his ex-wife and two young children. Twenty years later, in 1975, the Secretary of the Army contacted Blauer's daughters about a press release identifying the army's involvement in their father's death.[7] Finally, in 1987, a court awarded Blauer's daughters $702,044 in compensation from the federal government.

At around the same time that the Blauer case began in the early 1950s, the Atomic Energy Commission was helping to support studies that would demonstrate the peaceful uses of nuclear energy (Grodin, 1992). In one such episode that came fully to light only a few years ago, the AEC co-sponsored with the Quaker Oats

5. Blauer was aware that the drugs he was given were "experimental" in the sense that they did not come off the shelf of a pharmacy; however, the primary purpose of the experiment was to gather data that the Chemical Corps required for its investigation of the mescaline derivatives as potential chemical warfare agents.
6. The court issued findings of fact and conclusions of law that stated that Blauer had died as a result of New York State's negligence.
7. Blauer's eldest daughter filed an administrative claim with the Department of the Army for wrongful death of her father. She filed action in federal court in 1976.

company a study of mineral intake in the human body, using as a tracer minute amounts of radiation in breakfast cereal. Research subjects included emotionally disturbed adolescent boys in Massachusetts institutions known as Fernald and Wrenthem. At Fernald, about which more is known than Wrenthem, parents were asked to consent for their boys' participation in a special program called the "science club." They were not told the true purpose of the club, nor that they would be ingesting tiny amounts of radiation. In its 1995 Final Report to the President, the Advisory Committee on Human Radiation Experiments found that government officials and biomedical professionals even *at that time* "should have recognized that when research offers *no prospect* of medical benefit, whether subjects are healthy or sick, research should not proceed without the person's consent" (Grodin, 1992).[8]

Both the Blauer and Fernald-Wrenthem cases involved decisionally impaired subjects. The experiments were intended neither to benefit the subjects nor to address the conditions that caused their impairments. Interestingly, both projects were at least partly sponsored by national security agencies, a sector of government that used mental patients in research during the Second World War (Rothman, 1994). The vast majority of wartime subjects were military personnel (mainly in mustard gas studies), conscientious objectors, or prisoners. Psychotic patients were used in a malaria study, and retarded subjects participated in dysentery vaccine experiments sponsored by the Committee on Medical Research, an arm of the Executive Office of the President.

Within the array of more commonly cited research ethics scandals, there is one that also falls into the category of research with the decisionally impaired that is neither intended to benefit them directly nor contribute to knowledge about the condition that caused their decisional impairment. In the infamous Brooklyn Jewish Chronic Disease Hospital case in 1963, debilitated patients were injected with live cancer cells, apparently without their knowledge (Faden and Beauchamp, 1986). The study's purpose was to gather information on how the systems of patients with noncancerous chronic conditions would respond to the presence of trans-

8. Emphasis in the original.

planted cells. The investigators claimed to have obtained verbal consent of some sort from the subjects and defended the lack of documentation on the grounds that more dangerous procedures than this one were performed without consent forms and that they did not want to frighten the patients. When complaints were filed, state regulatory agencies responded with unusual vigor, and the principle investigator was censured by the New York State Board of Regents, which at that time was responsible for physician certification in the state (Katz et al., 1972).

HISTORIC REGULATORY EFFORTS

Most efforts to regulate the use of human subjects have been stimulated by concerns for children in research, likewise, but to a lesser extent, for pregnant women and fetuses, and later, for prisoners. Nonetheless, prior to the 1970s there were some widely scattered attempts to apply guidelines to the experimental use of the decisionally impaired. One of these occurred in Weimar, Germany. In 1930 a Jewish doctor named Julius Moses reported that seventy-five children had died in Lubeck as a result of pediatricians' experiments with a tuberculosis vaccine (Grodin, 1992). The German press was highly critical of the powerful chemical manufacturers for using hospitals to test their new products. The scandal in Lubeck gave substance to the accusations that people were being exploited for potential profits.

It happened that Moses was also a member of the German Parliament from the Social Democratic Party. In 1931 he played a key role in pressuring the Interior Ministry to respond to the Lubeck scandal (Grodin, 1992). The resulting rules were far more comprehensive and sophisticated than anything introduced by any government until then, and they compare quite favorably with modern regulations. They included a requirement for consent from informed human subjects. Like so much progressive government in the ill-fated Weimar Republic, these regulations were trampled by Hitler's regime, which used tens of thousands of concentration camp inmates in vicious experiments. After the war, at the Nuremberg trial of the Nazi doctors in 1947, the prosecution team alleged the use of the Interior Ministry guidelines as evidence that these prior standards should have governed the actions of the Hitler regime in the use of human experimental subjects. As a counter-argument, the legal status of the 1931 guidelines was questioned because they were not cited by the international organization that monitored public health laws and regulations in the 1930s and 1940s.

The team that investigated the Nazi crimes took notice of the abuse of the mentally ill in the context of the "T-4" or "euthanasia" program[9] that led to the extermination of many psychiatric patients and was, in effect, a rehearsal for the mass murders in the concentration camps (Proctor, 1992). The chief medical advisor to the Nuremberg judges, Leo Alexander, made the Nuremberg prosecutions possible by unraveling the horrific story of the camp experiments from the records of SS chief Heinrich Himmler (Grodin, 1992). Near the end of the trial, Alexander wrote a memorandum to the judges, portions of which were incorporated into the famous Nuremberg Code (Procter, 1992; U.S. Dept. of Energy, 1993). His memorandum became a part of the judges' decision that was their attempt to establish rules to guide human experimentation (Grodin, 1992). He also singled out the mentally ill as a population that should be given special protections. The judges deleted this reference in their final draft. A likely explanation is that they did not want to appear to be interfering in legitimate medical judgments about innovative treatment, but only to rule out nonbeneficial and highly risky experiments with easily coerced populations of healthy subjects as prisoners. Even so, much confusion about the judges' intentions has been caused by the Nuremberg Code's celebrated first line, that "the voluntary consent of the human subject is absolutely essential," a formulation that seems to rule out research with children, with emergency patients, and with the decisionally impaired.

When the National Commission for the Protection of Human Subjects of Biomedical and Behavioral Research was created in 1974 in the wake of the Tuskegee Syphilis Study scandal, the

---

9. The euthanasia program was planned and administered by the leaders of the German medical community after an October 1939 order issued from Hitler. The order required that certain doctors be commissioned to grant a "mercy death" to patients judged "incurably sick by medical examination." The gassing of the mentally ill was a rehearsal for the subsequent destruction of other "lives not worth living" (e.g., Jews, homosexuals, Communists, Gypsies, and prisoners of war).

decisionally impaired were not high on the list of special populations for consideration. The National Commission's report on
those "institutionalized as mentally infirm" (IMI) came at the very
end of their tenure in 1978. Moreover, in framing the topic in
terms of institutionalized persons, the report seemed to be obso-
lete. Movements toward de-institutionalization were already well
underway, if not largely completed, in many states. The coercive
aspects of institutionalization were familiar to the National Commission from its lengthy deliberations on prison research, but this
circumstance failed to capture the more subtle issues of study participation for persons who were no longer likely to be incarcerated
in "total institutions."

On its own terms, the National Commission's recommendations called for evaluating research with each class of IMI, including the mentally ill (*Protection of Human Subjects,* 43 Fed. Reg.,
1978). The commission found it advisable, in many instances, to
make use of a disinterested third party to ensure that the research
is not harmful. This individual might also play the role of a consent auditor, one who monitors the informed consent process itself and determines whether the potential subject has given a truly
competent consent. Tracking the framework used in its pediatric
recommendations, the National Commission also urged that persons with diminished capacity be allowed to "assent" to research
participation, after which their legally authorized representative
must be asked to consent on the subject's behalf.

There is remarkably little literature on the process that led to
the rejection of the National Commission's recommendations on
those institutionalized as mentally infirm in the early 1980s, although they were the least influential portion of the commission's
legacy. According to one former commission member and prominent bioethicist, Al Jonsen, officials at the National Institute of
Mental Health (NIMH) and the Agency for Drug Addiction and
Mental Health Association (ADAMHA) objected that the recommendations would stifle important research with their populations.[10] The reaction of the relevant professional community may

10. Interview with Al Jonsen, former member of the National Commission for the Protection of
Human Subjects of Biomedical and Behavioral Research (May 19, 1997).

perhaps be gauged from a paper published by a consultant to the commission, Harvard professor Neil Chayet, who argued in 1976 that the perspectives of law and medicine on informed consent are "fundamentally incompatible—particularly in the area of the mentally disabled, where appreciation of the concept of informed consent is well on its way to paralyzing research and treatment" (Chayet, 1976).

With the significant exception of the IMI recommendations, the 1981 Department of Health and Human Services rules largely followed the National Commission's work. In 1991 the rules were codified for seventeen federal agencies that conduct or sponsor research with human subjects and are now known as the "Common Rule" (*Protection of Human Subjects,* 45 C.F.R. 46.101–409, 1997). The regulations authorize institutional review boards (IRBs) to institute additional safeguards for research involving vulnerable groups, including the mentally disabled. The safeguards could involve consultation with specialists concerning the risks and benefits of a procedure for these populations, or special monitoring of consent processes to ensure voluntariness. But it is not known how frequently IRBs actually implement such further conditions.

THE CONTEMPORARY DEBATE

There is strong indirect evidence that IRBs are unlikely to compensate for the lack of specific regulations for research with the cognitively impaired by aggressive use of their discretionary authority. Observers of the local review process agree that if anything the IRB workload has greatly increased since the 1981 regulations were first implemented (U.S. Gen. Acct. Off., 1996). IRBs appear to have all they can handle to keep up with their paperwork as privately funded research has proliferated. Monitoring of a protocol's progress by IRBs after approval is practically nonexistent, apart from investigators' routine filing of annual progress reports. After the initial stages, the direct impact on actual research practices of local review is minimal.

The lack of specific federal guidance on research with the decisionally impaired has also meant that nonfederally funded research has gone its own way—or rather, at least fifty different ways. The states are a crazy quilt of regulation in this area, with most having no rules that clearly apply to this group, while some are quite restrictive (Hoffman and Schwartz, 1998). Recent events in the state of New York illustrate the situation. A state court has prohibited all state-sponsored greater-than-minimal-risk research with mental patients that does not hold potential benefit to the subjects. The decision in *T.D. v. New York State Office of Mental Health* (1996; 1997), resulting from a suit brought by former patients-subjects and several advocacy organizations, came with harsh criticism of state practices, some administrative, some technical, and some constitutional in nature.

It would be ironic if the lack of specific federal guidance resulted in even greater restrictions on research with the decisionally impaired than the National Commission contemplated. The commission's recommendations were virtually silent about what constitutes "benefit" to the subject, and what little was said about giving notice to subjects or permitting them to appeal research participation would not have satisfied the court in *T.D.*

The growing interest in research with the decisionally impaired stems partly from the most recent well-publicized incident with this population, the suicide of a former subject in a "drug free" or "washout" study at the University of California, at Los Angeles (Shamoo and Keay, 1996). Commentaries on this case and its implications often omit that the subject was two years out of the drug-free period of the study and one year out of observation from the study itself. Furthermore, the National Institutes of Health Office for Protection from Research Risks concluded that the study was ethical but that the informed consent form was flawed. Defenders of the research also claim that following admission to inpatient units, patients are often taken off all medication to establish a baseline, but withdrawing psychiatric drugs poses the danger of relapse and must be carefully managed (Baldessarini, 1978).

Several years after the controversy, how should the UCLA study be assessed? Often familiar accounts of ethics cases exaggerate the harms and wrongs done or the certainty that harms and wrongs were done. For example, the Willowbrook hepatitis studies, although they were ethically flawed, were more complicated in their ethical implications than is often appreciated (Beecher, 1970).[11] Similarly, as a former staff member of the President's Advisory Committee on Human Radiation Experiments, I have been surprised how often someone tells me how awful a certain radiation study was, when the committee had concluded that the case was far less terrible, or not clearly wrong, as compared to other problems, though not necessarily those that have attracted most of the attention. For example, how routine are drug holidays? Do studies that require a drug-free period simply "piggyback" on a common practice, or could the desire to enroll patients in studies determine the nature of their care? What merit is there to the theory that there is a "kindling" effect from repeated symptomatic episodes, so that subsequent psychotic states are exacerbated by previous ones? When provocation studies are conducted, should the return of symptoms associated with schizophrenia be evaluated as an inherent harm to be weighted against the potential for direct benefit to the patient?

It is a commonplace that the evolution of research ethics, and especially regulatory changes, is driven by scandal. The lack of guidance to IRBs in the current regulations and the flaws and inconsistencies in state laws would not, perhaps, have come to public attention had it not been for the *T. D.* case, which, if it does not rise to the level of scandal, has at least been a significant source of embarrassment and frustration to the New York psychiatric community. Accordingly, when President Clinton appointed the National Bioethics Advisory Commission in 1995, he included the review of current human subjects regulations in its mandate (Exec. Order No. 12,975). One population in which NBAC is especially interested is the decisionally impaired (NBAC, 1996).

It remains to be seen how the psychiatric and substance abuse treatment communities will react to any new recommendations that emerge from NBAC. It seems likely that whatever is brought

11. The Willowbrook study was "directed toward determining the period of infectivity of infectious hepatitis. Artificial induction of hepatitis was carried out in an institution for mentally defective children (many of whom were [five] to [eight] years old) in which a mild form of hepatitis was endemic. The parents gave consent for the intramuscular injection or oral administration of the virus, but little is said as to whether they were informed of the hazards involved" (Beecher, 1970).

forward will be perceived as more restrictive than the status quo, in that it will specify conditions for research with the decisionally impaired. However, psychiatric research has changed a great deal in the past twenty years. Those who conduct pharmacologic and biologic research are more accustomed to regulation than were those who performed behavioral research twenty-five years ago, and the former are now dominant in psychiatry.

TOWARD REGULATORY REFORM

There may be few instances of actual abuse in contemporary research involving those who are decisionally impaired. Unfortunately, there is no systematic study of this question. What is clear is that many, but by no means all, advocates for this group believe that more specific rules are needed. However, they are also loathe to impose restrictions that would significantly retard medical progress. As Alexander Capron (1997) has recently written, "no type of research raises more problems than research with the mentally impaired, particularly those who are institutionalized for treatment." Yet among populations that are often regarded as "vulnerable" and in need of special protection, persons who are decisionally impaired stand out as potential subjects for whom no regulations have been tailored.

In general terms, there have been many changes in the medical research environment since the 1981 enactment of the Department of Health and Human Services regulations (56 Fed. Reg. 28,002) that in 1991 were codified as the "Common Rule" for seventeen federal agencies (45 C.F.R. 46.101–404). Among the most important of these changes are the increase in multi-site studies and the increasing proportion of privately funded research (U.S. Gen. Acct. Off., 1996). As a result, IRBs are faced with challenges not contemplated two decades ago. They are often in an awkward position with regard to changes in consent forms for important and lucrative multi-site studies, and they are ill-equipped to monitor their colleagues' potential conflicts of interest in contract research. The increasing workload for IRBs has not been accompanied by increased resources for their support, and as presently structured, the Office for Human Research Protections (OHRP) has little discretion to alter regulatory requirements and encourage a more activist role for IRBs while relieving them of some paperwork that could be handled by qualified staff. Finally, there is growing congressional concern about research that does not come under federal informed consent requirements, either because it is privately funded or because the sponsors do not plan to pursue FDA approval for a drug or device (Satcher, 1997).

This litany of general comments about likely areas of continued discussion applies, of course, to research with those who are decisionally impaired as well. But there are a number of more specific items concerning this population. Each of them could be a discussion in itself.

First, a lively debate is beginning about the suitability and practicality of advance research directives for those who are able to anticipate a substantial period of decisional impairment. These directives may be procedural (durable powers-of-attorney for health care) or substantive (specifying what unapproved treatment may be attempted and under what circumstances), but they may be limited by at least two factors, current state laws and practicality (Karlawish and Sachs, 1997).

Second, if advance research directives are found to be ethically and legally acceptable and practical, it will need to be determined whether interventions not intended to benefit the patient, or those bearing more than a minor risk, may be authorized in advance by the potential subject. As Rebecca Dresser and Peter Whitehouse (1997) have recently argued, "Determining an acceptable balance of risks and potential benefits is the most important ethical challenge in emergency and nonemergency research involving decisionally incapable subjects."

Third, the National Commission's earlier suggestion about utilizing "consent auditors" (Dresser and Whitehouse, 1997) during the recruitment of decisionally impaired potential subjects may have renewed prospects. Not only would this system provide another layer of accountability with a disinterested third party, but if required for certain kinds of research, it would serve to encourage IRBs to do more active monitoring of consent processes. Consent auditors might also contribute to the education of investigators and their team members with regard to the conditions for a valid consent.

Fourth, the medical community is going to have to accept the need to subject certain popular study designs to greater scrutiny. "Washout" studies are a prime example, both because of the direct harm that is done to subjects by the return of symptoms and because of the indirect harm that may be associated with burdensome procedures conducted during the drug-free period, such as the use of neurological imaging devices that can entail discomfort and distress (Appelbaum, 1996). It may still be possible to conduct such studies by making certain modifications, such as beginning a trial with the most moderately affected patients.

Fifth, notice of entrance into a study, as was mentioned previously, should be required, regardless of capacity, with an appeals process built into the system. As the Maryland Working Group has suggested in its draft legislative proposal, prima facie dissent by the subject, regardless of capacity, must be clearly identified in the future as an absolute bar to further participation (Schwartz, 1998). A related but more difficult question is whether periodic "re-consenting" should be required for certain subjects at certain times in the study, including those subjects whose conditions may render them especially compliant due to dependency (Dresser, 1996).

Finally, the FDA's "narrow exception" to the informed consent requirement for emergency research (21 U.S.C. 355i)[12] may someday be used to justify consent waivers for nonemergency research that is hypothesized to present a very favorable risk-benefit ratio. This movement will begin with those whose decisional impairment is acute and who can be retrospectively "consented" within hours or perhaps days of the intervention. Attempts will then be made to extend the exception to those whose decisional impairment is chronic and whose capacity to consent is a distant possibility. It is not too early to consider whether any system can adequately protect subjects from inappropriate applications of such

12. "Such regulations shall provide that such exemption shall be conditioned upon the manufacturer, or the sponsor of the investigation, requiring that experts using such drugs for investigational purposes . . . that they will inform any human beings to whom such drugs . . . are being administered . . . that such drugs are being used for investigational purposes and will obtain the consent of such human beings or their representatives, except when they deem it not feasible or, in their professional judgment, contrary to the best interests of such human beings."

arrangements or whether a barrier must be constructed against further consent waivers.

APOLOGIA

I am a philosopher, not a physician; a critic, not an investigator. Confined to taking potshots from the sidelines, I will never enjoy credit for the medical advances that will someday brighten the lives of those who are decisionally impaired.

For nearly twenty years my father took care of a young man from a middle-class family in New Jersey, a man I will call Sam. When Sam arrived at my father's hospital in 1949, he was depressed and withdrawn. After several years of institutionalization he had improved, and his family prevailed upon my father to let him go home for a long weekend. A foolish uncle, thinking that Sam must need some masculine "R&R," took Sam to a prostitute. He was unable to perform, and he returned to the hospital in a profoundly depressed state that progressed to a psychosis from which he never recovered. For many years he lived in the bucolic setting of my father's sanitarium in a room that was sparsely furnished so that he could not hurt himself. A man whose robust physique contained a gentle spirit and a painfully vulnerable person, Sam was cared for meticulously by nurses and attendants. He expressed himself mainly through high-pitched whines and bleating sounds that I will never forget. My childhood friends, upon first hearing Sam's ranting while we played on the grounds, were shocked, then curious, but quickly grew accustomed to the unworldly conversations that took place deep within Sam's soul.

Guilt-ridden, my father was determined not to repeat his earlier mistake and grew fiercely protective of his patient. An old-fashioned psychiatrist who would surely be characterized as paternalistic by later bioethicists like me, he feared the abuses to which Sam would be exposed in a state hospital. For several years there was only one patient in the old sanitarium building in the Hudson Valley. Finally, when my father was nearly 80 years old, the insurance premiums became too expensive, and he had to give up his state license. The day of Sam's transfer was one of the saddest days that I remember in our household.

The LSD experiments on the decisionally impaired were speculative and perhaps risky, but there was nothing abstract about Sam's illness or the suffering it caused him and his family. Surely medical research with persons who are decisionally impaired must continue. How it is to be done without undermining the very humanity it seeks to promote will always entail an exquisitely delicate balance.

PART FOUR

THE MEANINGS OF NUREMBERG

The two most influential documents in the history of medicine are the Hippocratic Oath and the Nuremberg Code. They are also among the least read and most cited documents in the history of medicine. Considering that they are both so short and so widely available, it is remarkable that people refer to them so much and read them so little.

At least of the Oath it can be said that generations of scholars have pored over it and striven to comprehend it in its context. The same cannot be said for the Code, which is, after all, not even sixty years old. A tradition of scholarship as concerns the Code is only now getting established. I was fortunate to become part of this tradition when I worked for the President's Advisory Committee on Human Radiation Experiments in 1994–95. The committee's charge was to find the facts concerning decades of federally sponsored experiments with ionizing radiation and to determine whether they were conducted in accord with historic and current ethical conventions. We worked hard for a too-brief eighteen months and issued a 1,000-page report in a fairly small font.

One of my jobs was to reconstruct the American national security establishment's policies and practices concerning human experiments since 1945, and especially in the critical post–World War II period. Many of the documents with which I worked were declassified for the committee. I was given a top secret clearance so that I could view thousands of items to determine whether they should be put on a fast track to declassification. It was a dream job for an archives groupie.

A set of documents that I was the first to read was transcripts of meetings of Pentagon advisory committees in the late 1940s and early 1950s. I could hardly believe what I read. They told an amazing story about the defense department's struggles at the beginning of the cold war to develop a human experiments policy that was consistent with their needs for scientific information as the crisis with the Soviet Union and "Red China" erupted. Still more fascinating was the fact that these advisors felt constrained to worry about the propriety of doing potentially risky experiments, especially in the wake of the trials of Nazi doctors. Although there were few explicit references to the Nuremberg court, it was clear that the potential for drawing analogies was not far from their minds. The first chapter in this part reconstructs these debates and their peculiar outcome, using excerpts from the transcripts themselves.

The following chapter probes the reaction of the medical community to the Code and the revelations of Nazi medical crimes. Viewed through the notoriously unreliable "retrospectorscope" (a concept familiar to medical students), it would seem only natural that the Code would have had a tremendous influence on American medicine and our experimental practices. But the evidence indicates that the Code had little effect, as I explain. A set of rules developed in the wake of Nazi atrocities hardly seemed relevant to us. Only as we have looked back to rewrite our history has the Code assumed the influence and wisdom that we now commonly attribute to it.

10

"The Only Feasible Means":

The Pentagon's Ambivalent Relationship

with the Nuremberg Code

In the early 1950s, advisory committees in the U.S. Department of Defense (DOD) engaged in highly classified discussions about the permissible use of human subjects in military research. In spite of grave reservations expressed by many military officers and physician consultants, Pentagon officials not only adopted a formal set of rules to govern these activities, but they settled upon using the Nuremberg Code verbatim, making it even more rigorous with the addition of a requirement for written consent of subjects. Subsequently, however, the Pentagon policy was accorded limited influence not only in the defense establishment but also among physician-investigators who were DOD contract researchers.

This strange and rich story has been largely unknown to medical historians and philosophers. A few commentators have alluded to the Pentagon policy in the bioethics literature (Annas and Grodin, 1992), but only recently has it become possible to place the document in historical context. Previous work on this subject has been limited by the classified status of many of the background documents and the complexity of the story in which they are embedded.

But on 15 January 1994, President Clinton created the Advisory Committee on Human Radiation Experiments (ACHRE). The committee was charged with uncovering the history of these experiments and of the intentional releases of radiation, identifying the ethical and scientific standards for judging them, and recommending ways to ensure that any wrongdoing could not be repeated. Along with the executive order that created the committee, the president also ordered a massive declassification process throughout the federal bureaucracy of any material that would shed light on this story.

As a member of the committee staff, I was charged with poring over thousands of once-secret documents that might help tell the story of the evolution of federal standards in relation to the use of human subjects.[1] Especially critical was the tense decade following World War II, characterized by the early cold war, the Korean War, and McCarthyism. How did government advisors and policymakers weigh considerations of national security and human rights in this extraordinary time?

MOTIVATIONS FOR POLICY CREATION AFTER WORLD WAR II

Following the end of World War II there was a perceived need at the highest levels of the defense establishment for information from human experiments. This perception stemmed from two sources. First, it was believed that the Soviet Union was engaged in an intensive research and development program not only in conventional weapons but also in atomic, biological, and chemical warfare. Since the late 1940s Pentagon defense planners and scientists had begun to learn from human "experiments of opportunity." These included several radiation accidents among Manhattan Project laboratory workers, the mass exposures at Hiroshima and Nagasaki, and the frustrating clean-up effort following the underwater detonation at Operation Crossroads in 1947. In

---

1. Like some other committee and staff members, I was granted a "top secret" security clearance so that I could inspect other potentially relevant documents and, as needed, recommend that they be put on a "fast track" for declassification.

particular, the Crossroads experience impressed war planners with the insidious nature of radiation hazards, hazards that are invisible and therefore hard for military commanders to manage. Panic reactions among both civilian populations and armed forces personnel were considered perhaps the greatest single threat posed by atomic warfare, and they could be studied only with human subjects. A desire began to emerge for more controlled experiments to explore such matters (ACHRE, 1996).

Also in this period, radiation safety concerns shifted from laboratory workers to military personnel. Along with the widespread assumption that World War III was soon to be fought was the notion that it would take place on an atomic battlefield. Therefore, it was important not only to prepare combatants for the experience of nuclear warfare but also to understand how best to protect them from radiation effects so that they could be maximally effective as fighters in such an environment, and how to treat them for the ill-effects of exposures. Another major concern was how to protect and care for noncombatants who were at high risk of exposure in an era of "total war." Radiobiologists had long accepted the view that there is a threshold of acceptable exposure; defense planners needed to know what that threshold was and how field medicine could best respond if that exposure were exceeded. Some planners explicitly expressed less concern about long-term effects of radiation, which would not, of course, hinder troop battlefield performance. Several surveys of health physicists and others expert in radiation biology at that time produced wildly disparate estimates of permissible doses, a matter of considerable frustration to military officials.

Similar issues were raised by biochemical warfare research. In December 1951, for example, the secretary of defense expressed concern in a DOD directive about "our lack of readiness in chemical and biological warfare," and ordered the three services to increase their activities in these areas (Secretary of Defense, 1951).[2]

2. This and all subsequently referenced documents gathered by the Advisory Committee are on deposit in Record Group 220 (Presidential Committees, Commissions, and Boards) at the National Archives and Records Administration, Washington, D.C. Whenever possible, I have provided specific record identifiers from the ACHRE document collection system. Unfortunately, many of the documents cited were processed and assigned "ACHRE numbers" after I worked on them. It is my hope that future scholars will be able to retrieve the relevant documents based on the information I am able to provide in the citations.

Similarly, a joint meeting of representatives of all three service branches was held on 11 February 1952 to discuss "increased emphasis on CW and BW" (chemical and biological warfare). The minutes of that meeting include the summary statement: "That we have a serious need for increased testing of these weapons, in particular, experiments involving humans" (Department of Defense, 1952a). Reporting on these meetings to the secretary of defense on 25 April 1952, the assistant for special security programs emphasized the problem by stating: "If the signal to retaliate were given tomorrow, or even within the next year, the United States could make little more than a token effort" (Assistant Secretary for Special Security Problems, 1952). To concerns about what might be called the "biochem gap" were gradually added similar worries about radiation preparedness, and by sometime in 1952 all three areas were routinely considered together as "ABC warfare research."

Thus, a union of national security, scientific, and medical concerns emerged in this period, along with the view of many national security officials that human experiments were necessary. Yet defense planners also appreciated that human experimentation had unsavory associations in the public mind. The revelations of Nazi crimes and the Nuremberg doctors' trial did nothing to assuage such suspicions, and Pentagon medical advisory committees evidenced in their deliberations some awareness of the importance of these events for policymaking. At the same time, it was also widely believed that there was no moral similarity between what the Americans were contemplating and the Nazis' exploitation of concentration camp inmates. Nuremberg appears to have exercised both moral and public relations constraints on Pentagon officials and advisors; the question that divided many, especially between 1950 and 1952, was what the appropriate response should be to these constraints.

To be sure, there were also legal concerns about human experimentation in the DOD at mid-century. Fear of suit by aggrieved service personnel was probably not the primary motivation for these concerns, since that kind of action was significantly less likely even to be seriously considered than is the case today. Rather, difficult insurance questions arose concerning indemnification of civilian volunteers in case of injury related to an experiment. Military personnel were automatically covered for injuries incurred during service, and at this time the armed forces did not require that experiment volunteers from the ranks give up their rights to be compensated (ACHRE, 1996).

Finally, DOD administrators were engaged in an extensive reorganization process in the early 1950s. During that process it became evident that the Pentagon lacked the technical authority to conduct human experiments according to its own operating policies, experiments that many defense planners thought highly desirable. This is not to suggest that the defense department was not conducting medical experiments involving human subjects during this period, but the controversial new experiments that were proposed impelled the department to develop a more formal policy. In a memo dated 5 February 1953, the director of the executive office of the secretary of defense wrote of proposed atomic, biological, and chemical warfare, experiments: "There is no DOD policy on the books which permits this type of research" (Underwood, 1953). Thus, the lack of a rules on human experiments became another important impetus to introduce some kind of formal policy. More difficult was just what kind of policy to introduce.

THE ROBERT S. STONE CONTROVERSY

A paper by Robert S. Stone, M.D., dated 31 January 1950, apparently formed the basis of a discussion within the office of the secretary of defense about conducting human experiments that would make it possible to predict the biological effects of radiation exposure (Stone, 1950).[3] This discussion is a window into the themes and tensions that suffused this question. Stone was

---

3. It is evident that the Navy and the Joint Panel on Medical Aspects of Atomic Warfare (which included AEC and DOD representatives) favored the use of human subjects at this time, while the Army and the Committee on Medical Sciences of the Pentagon's Research and Development Board did not. This episode is also covered in Gilbert Whittemore, "A Crystal Ball in the Shadows of Nuremberg and Hiroshima: The Ethical Debate over Human Experimentation to Develop a Nuclear Powered Bomber, 1946–1951," in *Science, Technology and the Military* (1988), pp. 431–62. A propos the present paper, Whittemore observes that "ethical arguments may be much more common [in high level national security debates] than one would judge from published material alone" (p. 432).

professor of radiology at the University of California at San Francisco and a member of the Nuclear Energy Propulsion for Aircraft (NEPA) Medical Advisory Committee. His nine-page paper is a systematic and scholarly defense of the proposition that human radiation testing is needed and that it is ethical. Not only the nuclear-powered aircraft then being researched but also the prospect that soldiers and sailors would be exposed to radiation from weapons as a result of international hostilities formed the strategic basis of the need argument. From a scientific standpoint, Stone noted the wide disagreement among radiologists about dosages that would produce "specific effects" in humans. Thus, Stone recommended that some people be exposed to 25 r (roentgens) and observed. If there were no "significant" changes, then the dosage should be doubled, and then repeated a week later. If there were again no significant changes, the amount should be at least doubled. Based on experience with sick patients at these levels, Stone writes, "It seems unlikely that any particular person would realize that any damage had been done to him by such exposure." Stone argued that the small risks of "undetectable genetic effect" on the life span or possibly on the blood must be weighed against the advantages of actual human exposure, such as reassuring pilots who would carry out a particular mission.

Stone noted that the use of human subjects in medical experiments was not new, citing Jenner's development of a smallpox vaccine, Walter Reed's yellow fever work, the use of federal prisoners by the Public Health Service, and armed forces research on malaria with Illinois state prisoners. In a section entitled "The Ethics of Human Experimentation," Stone cited Dr. Andrew Ivy's well-known article published in *Science* in July 1948. Dr. Ivy was a medical ethics advisor to the Nuremberg judges, and in his article he states that the most important ethical requirement is that subjects be volunteers who are under no "undue pressure" to participate. Stone also cited the American Medical Association's code of ethics and the analysis of a committee appointed by Governor Dwight H. Green of Illinois (chaired by Dr. Ivy) concerning the use of prisoners as experimental subjects, published in *JAMA* February 1948.

Stone concluded that the proposed radiation experiments met all ethical criteria, and he recommended that a subject population be identified that could be followed years after exposure: "Life prisoners are the one group of people that are likely to remain in one place where they can be observed for a great many years." To obtain "short term results," other types of subjects might be used. "Patients with incurable cancer such as those having multiple metastases might volunteer. . . . Certain scientists might be willing to volunteer for specific doses" as well as some in the "general population," but again, they might be hard to follow. Those under 21 should be ruled out because they cannot legally volunteer, and "those below the menopause (unless they have incurable cancer) probably should not be used because of psychological factors." The advantages and disadvantages of these two populations for research purposes would be revisited time and again in secret discussions.

Stone's paper generated considerable reaction in the DOD and in the Atomic Energy Commission (AEC) during the following months. For example, at the Pentagon's Committee on Medical Sciences meeting on 31 January–1 February 1950, the members were deeply split on the question of human experiments. Some appeared to support the view that there was a need for human experiments under "safe" conditions using "volunteers," and others were clearly opposed to any such studies. The following exchanges are representative not only of the division within the committee on this issue but also of the breadth of the subjects covered and the uncertainty among many members about the right approach to take (Department of Defense, 1950).[4]

> Dr. Fenn [Dr. Wallace O. Fenn, University of Rochester]: Mr. Chairman, I'd like to say a word about human experimentation because I have a feeling that is a very dangerous route to get started on and that we shouldn't sanction human experimentation without careful consideration. . . . I think we will get the information that is required from animals, animal experimen-

---

4. Identifications are based on information provided in the documents themselves; further information is not always available.

tation and accidental exposure and shouldn't approve routine experimentation on volunteers. I'd like to hear some discussion about it.

GEN. ARMSTRONG [Maj. Gen. Harry C. Armstrong, U.S. Air Force Medical Corps]: I don't believe we can adopt that stand because if we do it for that we should do it for all areas of research, and certainly, many of our valuable findings in the past have been based on volunteer human experimentation. I think that the actual research should be evaluated in each individual case and certainly given every possible safeguard, but if we go on record as being opposed to human research experimentation in this field we should apply it, I believe, to all fields.

DR. FENN: I wouldn't make it quite as broad as that. I'd qualify that a little.

GEN. ARMSTRONG: I don't see there is any great difference in principle in undertaking a hazardous procedure. It seems to me it doesn't make much difference whether it's an atomic energy or using an ejection seat at 530 miles an hour. They are both likely to kill you, and I don't see any particular reason why we should include any area, or if you include one you must include them all, I don't see where you should make any distinction.

DR. BLAKE [Dr. Francis G. Blake, Chairman]: In individual cases it comes down to assessment of risk, doesn't it?

GEN. ARMSTRONG: That's right. I certainly don't think we should advocate widespread and superficial plunging into this thing by any means, but I don't think we can solve that by simply saying we are not in favor of any human experimentation.

Contrasting with the ambivalence within the DOD was the reaction of the advisory committee of the AEC's Division of Biology and Medicine in their meeting of 8 and 9 September 1950. The committee recorded its opposition to human experiments "at the present time," noting also "serious repercussions from a public relations standpoint if undertaken by an agency that has to do a portion of its work in secret" (Atomic Energy Commission, 1950a).

The Pentagon's Committee on Medical Sciences met again on 23 May 1950. This time they considered a proposal to use "long-term prisoners" as subjects for the radiation research. There was agreement that, if this were to be done, the studies would have to be in conformity with the research principles adopted by the AMA in December 1946. The author of these rules, Dr. Andrew Ivy, was also the AMA's advisor on the Nuremberg prosecution of medical war criminals and an expert witness at the trial. The Nuremberg tribunal evidently used his memorandum to the AMA as the basis for much of the language contained in the Nuremberg Code. Although published in small print in *JAMA* in 1946 as part of other association business ("Supplemental report of the judicial council," 1946), the AMA's formal position was well known enough to be part of a Pentagon committee's conversation.

A fascinating debate ensued in the Committee on Medical Sciences that day about whether long-term prisoners or cancer patients being treated with radiation therapy would be more appropriate subjects, considering the questions at issue (Department of Defense, 1950b).

> ADMIRAL GREAVES [Rear Adm. F. C. Greaves, Medical Corps, U.S. Navy]: I agree with Colonel Stone in that there certainly is a need for this type of information, particularly in view of the fact that we are going to be confronted with the problem of protecting personnel, not only in airplanes, but also in submarines, of this type of thing . . . But this is a long-range thin[g], and people who have types of diseases in which it is necessary to give them x-ray therapy may not be with us long enough to make the information we get valid.
>
> COL. STONE [This is a different person from Dr. Robert S. Stone, mentioned above]: Admiral Greaves, I'd like to point out that from the Army's viewpoint, at least, the levels that we are particularly interested in are those of relatively short duration. In other words, a man may develop a cancer twenty years later but if he is in the middle of combat we don't think that would actually deter from actually something [*sic*], so that what we are interested in is what level is going to make this man sick or noneffective within a period of thirty days, in all probability. Now we are very much interested in long-term effects, but when you start thinking militarily of this, if men are going out on these missions anyway, a high percentage is not coming back, the fact that you may get cancer twenty years later is just of no significance to us.

DR. COGGESHALL [Dr. Lowell T. Coggeshall]: What about the other way around? Do you believe you get answers from people subject to radiation therapy usually by reason of neoplastic disorders?

COL. STONE: I think it would have to be a selective study. For instance, take any of our big centers where we have quite a lot of cases of carcinomas (you can't pick lymphomas, but carcinomas types of metastasis); a number of those individuals will live in varied states of health from a period of six to eight months and x-ray therapy was indicated in epilating measures [doses sufficient to cause hair loss], and I think when we study our material on the population in Japan, plus our combined animal work, then we might logically draw up a series of bracketing experiments in which you probably get thirty to fifty such cases in a hospital like Memorial Hospital, for instance, in New York, or certain hospitals in other cities, by carefully selecting the cases and getting the amount of radiation from that bracket we might be able to get a very satisfactory answer.

ADM. GREAVES: I agree with that absolutely. We could use information from whatever source, but I am wondering if we are not being a little too skiddish [sic] about this. We have a problem on our hands and I think we should consider it very seriously, but whether it is enough of a problem to go ahead and take a chance . . .

COL. STONE: Well, we think it is a problem, all right, and certainly willing [sic] to take a chance on this thing. It is a question about whether you are going to get the best information in the most scientific manner . . .

COL. DECOURSEY [Col. Elbert DeCoursey, Medical Corps, U.S. Army]: . . . I must say that in my own mind I realize that all of these things are important to know and we must know them, but it is difficult for me to come to a decision of whether or not you should go into human experimentation on this because of the world opinion on the experimentation in Germany. That bothers me.

ADM. GREAVES: I find it very difficult too.

DR. FENN: . . . I question, myself, whether the end is going to justify the means. We certainly ought to do every other method until we are absolutely certain it can't give us any information. I think the important thing is whether you take the decision to go down this road of human experimentation and work on prisoners, even though they are volunteers, and start the idea that as long as they are prisoners it really doesn't matter very much what you do to them, and it is no great loss to society, which I think it isn't, but it is a bad decision.

DR. COGGESHALL: I'd say, in comment on this, they are already down this road. There is quite a bit of human utilization of prisoners, of one type or another. It seems to me it differs only in the type of work they propose to do, not in the opinions of the thing. That doesn't make it right, necessarily, but . . . [ellipses in transcript].

ADM. GREAVES: I think the reasoning behind the proposal to use prisoners was that they are long-term prisoners and that they would be available for observation and study. I don't think the reason for the proposal to use prisoners is because they were prisoners to society, or little use to society. The reason was that they would be there and you can put your finger on them and observe them for a long period of time. That isn't true of volunteers from the rest of the world, either Armed Forces or otherwise. They are here maybe this year and gone next. You lose track of them. This is a long-term thing.

The proposal was referred to the Armed Forces Medical Policy Council (AFMPC), a body that subsequently played an important role in the promulgation of the draft human experiments policy, on 30 June 1951. The issue of experimentation on human subjects was not confined to radiation studies but also had implications for research on biological and chemical warfare. On 17 December 1951 the AFMPC endorsed the principle that "final realistic evaluation of biological warfare must await appropriate field trials in which human subjects are used" (Department of Defense, 1951).

Sympathy for the view that human experimentation was unavoidable was growing. At its 8 September 1952 meeting, the AFMPC heard a presentation from the chief of preventive medicine of the army surgeon general's office concerning the medical services' role in the development of defensive measures and devices. "Following detailed discussion, it was unanimously agreed that the use of human volunteers in this type of research be approved" (Casberg, 1952). Interestingly, the proposition that human subjects were needed prevailed in the immediate context of biological and chemical, rather than radiation, experiments. What the debate did not provide (an explicit policy on human radiation experiments) would become available as an indirect result of worries about the future of biological and chemical weapons development.

ADOPTING THE NUREMBERG CODE

Now that human experimentation was accepted in principle, the problems of exactly what kind of rules should govern it remained. In October 1952 the AFMPC decided to adopt the ten rules of the Nuremberg Code, based on the advice of its legal counsel, Stephen S. Jackson, the Pentagon's assistant general counsel for manpower and personnel. Jackson also advised that there should be no exception for physicians who used themselves as subjects and that an eleventh rule should be added that explicitly prohibited experiments with prisoners of war (Jackson, 1952a).

It is hard to escape the conclusion that the decision to adopt the code was driven by legal reasons such as concern about insurance coverage in the event of injury to subjects, and that these kinds of concerns finally forced the issue, quite apart from the internal Pentagon debate that had been going on for several years. An extraordinary sentence from a letter written on 2 March 1953, the day it was learned that Eisenhower's new secretary of defense, Charles E. Wilson, had signed the memo, vividly documents Jackson's central role in crafting the DOD policy based on the Nuremberg Code:

> It was on Mr. Jackson's insistence that the "Nuremberg Principles" were used in toto in the document [the Wilson memo], since he stated, these already had international juridical sanction, and to modify them would open us to severe criticism along the line— "*see[,] they use only that which suits them*" [emphasis added]. (Rapalski, 1953)

The italicized passage in the above quotation is remarkable: a senior administration official in 1953 seems to have cited the 1947 ruling by the judges at the Nuremberg doctors' trial as setting international legal precedent to which American researchers should be held.

Jackson's superior, Anna M. Rosenberg, Assistant Secretary for Manpower and Personnel, was another important participant in drafting the ultimate proposal. Rosenberg was a nationally recognized authority on labor relations and had been an influential New Dealer. The highest-ranking woman to serve in the defense establishment up to that time, Rosenberg insisted that a further rule be added to the proposed policy, that "consent be expressed in writing before at least one witness" (Jackson, 1952b).

Several Pentagon medical advisory committees were then asked to comment on the draft proposal and gave it at best a cool reception. The Committee on Medical Sciences opposed any policy at all on the grounds that it "would probably do the cause more harm than good; for such a statement would have to be 'watered down' to suit the capabilities of the average investigator. Thus, it would be restrictive to the exceptional research worker" (Mussells, 1952). The committee also expressed the view that "human experimentation within the field of medical sciences has, in years past, and is at present an unwritten code of ethics" that is "administered informally" and "considered to be satisfactory. . . . To commit to writing a policy on human experimentation would focus unnecessary attention on the legal aspects of the subject."

At least one other DOD committee was engaged in the discussion and ultimately advanced an alternative recommendation. The Committee on Chemical Warfare, in its 10 November 1952 meeting, heard a draft of the Nuremberg Code–based proposal. After the reading one member remarked to general laughter, "If they can get any volunteers after that, I'm all in favor of it" (Department of Defense, 1952). The committee advanced an alternative proposal that a British-style system of rewards for volunteers should be employed. A consent form could then "be subject to the interpretation that uniformed volunteers could be assigned to temporary duty at the experimental installation for the purpose of engaging in the program as test subjects" (Worthley, 1952).

In spite of the reservations of these advisory committees, the AFMPC proposal had already been endorsed by general counsel and an assistant secretary. That top officials were committed to the eventual adoption of the Nuremberg Code-based draft is dramatically evidenced by a hand-written note from George V. Underwood, director of the executive office of the secretary of defense, to Deputy Secretary Foster dated 4 January 1953:

> I believe Mr. Lovett [secretary of defense under President Truman] has a considerable awareness of this proposed policy. It has been under development for some time. Because of the importance and controversial character of the policy, I strongly recommend advance clearance with Service Sec'ys [*sic*] thru Joint Sec'y's [*sic*] group. If you agree, we'd like to recapture the case so that copies can be made available to Service Sec'ys [*sic*].
>
> Since consequences of this policy will fall upon Mr. Wilson, it might be wise to pass [it] to him as a unanimous recommendation from the "alumni." (Underwood, 1953b)

A new administration was about to take power in Washington, and the top echelon of the Pentagon wanted to make sure that an important but controversial matter was placed before the new secretary of defense with all the support needed to make it easier for him to approve the proposed policy. To maximize support, the plan was to mobilize heavy artillery in the form of the service secretaries. But Underwood's plan failed. On 8 January 1953, Foster and the three service secretaries did not object but also were not enthusiastically favorable. One reason for this result might have been the absence of Secretary Lovett, who was testifying before Congress that day. It was decided only to refer the matter to Secretary Wilson because it was controversial, and in any case, it would be up to him to implement it if it were approved.

THE WILSON MEMORANDUM

In spite of the cool reception by other groups within the DOD, on 13 January 1953 the AFMPC's memo to the secretary of defense "strongly recommended that a policy be established for the use of human volunteers (military and civilian employees) in experimental research at Armed Forces facilities," and that such use "shall be subject to the principles and conditions laid down as a result of the Nuremberg Trials" (Casberg, 1953).

Finally, on 26 February 1953, the new secretary of defense did sign off on the proposed policy. His memorandum began with the following paragraph:

Based upon a recommendation of the Armed Forces Medical Policy Council, that human subjects be employed, under recognized safeguards, as the only feasible means for realistic evaluation and/or development of effective preventive measures of defense against atomic, biologic or chemical agents, that policy set forth below will govern the use of human volunteers by the Department of Defense in experimental research in the fields of atomic, biological and/or chemical warfare. (Secretary of Defense, 1953)

In the hustle and bustle of a new administration, it is unlikely that Secretary Wilson had very much time to consider the implications of the new policy on the use of human subjects, but he probably took it on faith that the AFMPC and the previous administration had done its homework. The memorandum was given the number TS-01188, "TS" standing for top secret (Secretary of Defense, 1953).

As the Pentagon's Committee on Medical Sciences began its meeting the next day, 27 February, they did not know about the new secretary's action. During a discussion of the potential harms of hepatitis studies, when it was mentioned that there had been three deaths in the Pentagon's program of prison studies, another remarkable debate about the use of human subjects took place (Department of Defense, 1953):

COL. WOOD [Col. John R. Wood, Medical Corps, U.S. Army, Army Chemical Center, Maryland]: I think if we have men volunteer who are satisfied that they are taking a full risk and they fully understand what this risk is, then we are justified in going ahead on the basis of absolute necessity and there being no alternative whatsoever. So I have mixed feelings about this thing. I would not be willing to be a volunteer. However, on the other hand, there is no other way to do this work.

CAPT. SHILLING [Capt. Shilling, M.D., Medical Corps, U.S. Navy]: In connection with the human volunteer problem in general, I think we have all discussed this for the last six months at all levels in the Department of Defense. There is one thing that disturbs me a great deal, and that is at the DOD level and at the Medical Policy Council Level [*sic*] there is a strong urge to try and set up an over-all policy for the conduct of human experimentation. They even go back to the Buchenwald trials, and they are trying to work [out] an over-all pattern that will, if you meet this pattern—To me, this is utterly fantastic as a method of approach.

As far as the Navy is concerned, I have cleared this with policy, and we want to strongly urge that human research be conducted as it is now outlined from a policy standpoint; namely, that the field or the individual or the groups who want to do the research prepare a complete experimental design, showing exactly what they want to do, what the safeguards are going to be, what the program is, why it has to be human rather than animal, and so forth, and then come in and be evaluated by the Surgeons General involved in the Army, Navy, and Air Force, and then that it go up to the Secretary informed for final permission. This is the way we do it now and I think we are going to get into a horrible mess if we try to set up an overall standard for every type of research. What happens is that you put so many safeguards on what we cannot do the multitude of things we are trying to do.

Moments later, the chair interrupted:

THE CHAIRMAN: We have here a document which was just brought in which is signed by Mr. Wilson, dated February 26th. With your permission, I would like to release this information. However, in order to do so, it will be necessary for any member of the audience to excuse himself if he does not have a top secret clearance.

After the letter was read to the committee, there was an off-the-record discussion of the new policy. Obviously, any further general objections to the policy were now academic.

The Wilson memo appears to represent a very high ethical standard in the spirit of the Nuremberg Code. But the standard is more limited than might at first be apparent. It is unclear, for example, how the policy was to apply to civilian contractors, or to those who are not normal volunteers (the population to which the Nuremberg Code seems limited) but individuals with active medical problems. These ambiguities were to be vexing in the future.

In the shorter term, the fact that the memorandum was at first top secret and only gradually downgraded prevented the new policy from being implemented as efficiently as it might have been, as we shall see. Some explanation for the top secret classification of the Wilson memo may be gleaned from the spirit of a 3 September 1952 memorandum from the secretary of the joint chiefs of staff to the joint chiefs; it also raises other questions about the determination of the military's interest in medical research conducted out of the public eye:

> 2. The Joint Chiefs of Staff further consider that responsible agencies should: . . . d. Insure, insofar as practicable, that all published articles stemming from the BW or CW research and development programs are disassociated from anything which might connect them with U.S. military endeavors. (Lalor, 1952)

WHY THE WILSON MEMO?

At least two interesting conclusions can be drawn about the process leading up to the Wilson memorandum. First, the idea of using the Nuremberg Code as the basis of a policy was received without enthusiasm among relevant advisory groups in the defense department. Second, apart from that reception, the question of what sort of policy the Pentagon should adopt concerning human experiments, and if they were needed at all, was a matter of vigorous debate even before the Wilson memo was presented in draft in 1952. This debate was further fueled when the draft policy was circulated.

Yet the debate that began at least as early as 1950 in the Pentagon was flawed. The protagonists spent most of their time staking out abstract philosophical positions for and against human experimentation in general. The real question, however, was not *whether* human experiments would take place (for human subjects were being used in medical research at that time, both inside and outside the military), but rather *how* human subjects may be used. There seems to have been little or no discussion of some basic questions: What is the meaning of "volunteering" once one is in the military? What are the limits of possible harm to which military personnel may acceptably be exposed? How can it be assured that no more individuals will be used in an experiment than are absolutely necessary?

Nor is there evidence, as yet, that those who promulgated the

Nuremberg Code as the basis of a policy understood its implications. Had this been the case, difficult questions would surely have been raised in anticipation of efforts to apply the code. The "controversy" about the use of human subjects and about the draft proposal that came out of the AFMPC thus largely missed the point. Interestingly, in spite of its lukewarm reception, the controversy behind it, and its potentially far-reaching consequences, the Nuremberg-like policy went from proposal to policy in a matter of months. Reading the documents, one has the sense that the poorly understood proposal had a momentum that was independent of the debate surrounding it and was certainly independent of the substance of the proposed policy. Indeed, the most reasonable explanation of its eventual formal success—and its ultimate practical limitations—is precisely that the Wilson memo grew out of the decision making of a few top officials of the Lovett defense department, especially the general counsel's office and Assistant Secretary Rosenberg, rather than out of the advisory process of internal experts on military medical research.[5]

It was the defense department's legal counsel and labor relations expert, not its physicians or defense planners, who seem to have originated and promoted the idea of using the Nuremberg Code and adding to it signed and witnessed consent as well as an explicit bar to the use of prisoners of war. And it was high officials in the office of the secretary of defense who carried it forward into the new administration. Members of the DOD upper echelon thus crafted a document that was state-of-the-art for the day, but not one that would enjoy the widespread allegiance of those who would have to implement it—or perhaps even the full understanding of those who promulgated it.

In a sense, the motivation of top officials to create a policy was straightforward: following the 1950 Department of Defense Reorganization Act, there was a perceived need for such a policy to cover the use of military personnel in experiments having to do with atomic, biological, and chemical warfare—experiments that were in turn regarded as imperative in the confrontation with the

5. This point was forcefully made by Jay Katz in our discussions during my work for the Advisory Committee.

Soviet Union. Human experiments involving "unconventional" forms of warfare, and especially radiation, were likely to be highly sensitive with the American public. Thus, the experiments being contemplated seemed to planners to fall into a different category as compared with more familiar kinds of military exercises or clinically based medical experiments.

This also explains why the comment process by Pentagon committees turned out to be largely a formality. For as the documents show, the office of the secretary of defense wanted to have some sort of policy on the books as soon as possible. The legal and personnel management impetus behind the draft proposal had its own raison d'être. But while the theory behind the Wilson memo triumphed in a formal sense, it did not settle the doubts among the officers and researchers who would have to live according to its rules. The military-medical bureaucracy's failure to embrace the memorandum's spirit was not a matter of insubordination, which would have been clear and relatively easy to manage; it was, rather, a matter of cultural resistance, and therefore far more subtle and difficult to control. It was perhaps for this reason more than any other, that the policy's consent requirements were at best sporadically applied in the two decades that followed.Indeed, not only the military establishment but American society as a whole only began to come to terms with the issues embodied in this debate nearly twenty-five years later in the mid-1970s, and then only after some highly publicized abuses of human subjects. In retrospect, it might be said that high Pentagon advisors and officials could hardly have been expected to resolve issues that continue to generate new and difficult questions following decades of further experience and reflection.

11

Reassessing the Influence of the Nuremberg
Code on American Medical Ethics

In this chapter I consider the role of the Nuremberg Code in
certain aspects of the evolution of research standards in the United
States. I argue that recent revelations about cold war deliberations
among high officials enable a far more nuanced understanding of
the code's role during the years following the war than had been
possible before this formerly classified material became available.

JUDGMENTS AT NUREMBERG

On August 19, 1947, the war crimes trials of twenty-three Nazi
physicians and bureaucrats in Nuremberg, West Germany, came
to a close. Known variously as *United States vs. Karl Brandt et al.,*
as the Nuremberg Medical Trial, or as the "Medical Case" (to
distinguish it from the trials of Nazi political, industrial, and military leaders), the trials began on December 9, 1946. The trials
took far longer than the prosecution expected, for the issues were
more complex than they appreciated at the outset, and the defense was able to exploit the fact that the conventions of human

subjects research were ambiguous, in spite of prosecution witnesses claims to the contrary. In the end, however, the three judges, all Americans, found fifteen of the defendants guilty of atrocities, sentencing seven to death.

The defense case apparently left a deep impression upon the Nuremberg judges. Rather than simply rule on the guilt or innocence of the defendants, they decided to formulate a set of statements that would leave no doubt about the ethical principles that must govern the use of human beings in medical science. In this effort they were strongly influenced by Dr. Andrew Ivy, an expert witness sent by the American Medical Association (AMA) to testify on medical ethics at the trials. Ivy had conducted experiments in the United States on questions similar to those pursued by the Nazi researchers, including seawater desalination and the effects of high altitudes, and had sometimes used human subjects.

In August 1946 Ivy prepared a 22-page document setting out the rules of human experimentation, giving one copy to the AMA's Judicial Council and another to the Nuremberg prosecutors. On December 11, 1946, the AMA House of Delegates approved a somewhat shorter version of Ivy's rules, which were subsequently published along with other items of business in the *Journal of the American Medical Association*. The most important provisions of the Nuremberg Code itself, which was published along with the rest of the tribunal's judgment in August 1947, reproduced verbatim most of Ivy's language, as well as two contributions from a memorandum prepared by the other American expert witness, Dr. Leo Alexander. The Code was also accompanied by the judges' assertion that these principles were already widely understood in the scientific community. Were that the case, a critic might wonder, then why was it necessary to formulate them in this context? Why would a simple declaration of guilt or innocence based on the facts of the matter not be sufficient?

THE NUREMBERG CODE IN THE UNITED STATES: THE STANDARD VIEW

Although the trials themselves were not, it seems, given close attention in the United States while they were going on, the guilty verdicts did make the front page of the *New York Times*. What, then, was the influence of the Nuremberg Code in the United States, especially in the years immediately following the trials? Several commentators have addressed this question. According to the standard view, the influence of the Code in the United States was virtually nil. As the historian David Rothman has put it, "The prevailing view was that [the Nuremberg defendants] were Nazis first and last; by definition nothing they did, and no code drawn up in response to them, was relevant in the United States" (Rothman, 1991, 63).

At least four reasons can be offered for the attitude summarized by Rothman. First, once the conduct of the Nazi doctors became known, it was regarded as so extreme and sui generis as to have little or no bearing on civilized people, who conducted scientific research according to the best lights of their consciences. Second, the concentration camps were regarded as a radically different environment from anything resembling a normal setting for medical studies, far more cruel even than a conventional prison. Third, the longstanding tradition of medical ethics, embodied in the Hippocratic Oath and in its beneficent philosophy, was regarded as a generally adequate basis upon which the medical profession could police itself. Fourth, the Code's absolute requirement for the "voluntary consent of the subject" was obviously inapplicable to populations upon whom important medical research was being done and had been done for some time, including children.

To be sure, there were some exceptions to this attitude. Although most popular press coverage of human subjects research was highly celebratory, there was the occasional critical article exposing the use of "human guinea pigs" in the years following World War II (O'Hara, 1948; Koritz, 1953). In the early 1950s, sociologist Renee Fox found that physician-scientists in a metabolic research ward were highly sensitive to the ethical dilemmas they faced, and she paraphrased the Nuremberg Code as the principle upon which the researchers she observed based their use of human subjects (Fox, 1974). But as Jay Katz has observed, for the most part the medical research community adopted the view that the Nuremberg Code was "a good code for barbarians but an unnecessary code for ordinary physicians" (Katz, 1996).

More pertinent to the territory staked out in this essay is the influence of the Nuremberg Code in the legal sphere. Leonard Glantz (1992) has argued that the Code has had little influence on federal regulations for the conduct of human subjects research, though his survey does not include the defense establishment, which is the focus here. George Annas has noted that the first U.S. court citation of the Code was in 1973, and concludes from his analysis of its subsequent career in court decisions that national security has generally trumped the Code in cases involving the abuse of human beings by defense-related federal agencies during the cold war (Annas, 1992).

Only once, in the case of *Stanley v. United States* (1987), has the U.S. Supreme Court commented on the use of the Code, and then only in dissent. In *Stanley*, an Army sergeant attempted to bring suit against the government for subjecting him to illegal drug experimentation, but his case was dismissed under the Feres doctrine, which prohibits members of the Armed Forces from suing the government for harms inflicted "incident to service."

In the remainder of this chapter, I reassess the influence of the Nuremberg Code on American medical ethics in the decade immediately following the Medical Trials, especially in the national security establishment. While my conclusion does not sharply differ from the standard view summarized above, more recent information suggests that the Code did have an influence in quarters that many would find surprising—not in the medical profession or research community itself, but in the councils of the national security establishment, as part of planning for defense against unconventional atomic, biological, and chemical weaponry. However, the Code's influence waned after the first decade following the war.

This reassessment is both justified and prompted by the Final Report of the President's Advisory Committee on Human Radiation Experiments, released by President Bill Clinton on October 3, 1995. The appointment of the ACHRE followed press reports of unethical experiments on human beings having been sponsored by federal agencies during the period 1944 to 1974, many in secret. These experiments included injecting hospitalized patients with plutonium, feeding radiation-laced breakfast cereal to institutionalized adolescents, exposing cancer patients to total-body irradiation, and irradiating the testicles of prisoners in state penitentiaries. In order to determine whether the experiments conformed to the ethical standards of the day or those now recognized, the Advisory Committee had unprecedented access to thousands of pages of formerly classified documents that related to the development of human research policies in the national security establishment. As a member of the ACHRE staff, I was charged with helping the committee come to an understanding of the nature and significance of these historical standards.

POSTWAR NOTICE OF NUREMBERG IN THE
ATOMIC ENERGY COMMISSION

In its investigation of the postwar period, the ACHRE found that there was a flurry of activity having to do with the use of human subjects in 1947 in the newly formed Atomic Energy Commission (AEC), the civilian entity that inherited many of the programs and contracts of the Manhattan Project. This activity was partly inspired by concern about a series of plutonium injections in hospitalized patients during the war that were apparently intended to help provide information about safe exposure levels to laboratory workers handling fission products. While the committee did not conclude that the AEC was directly influenced by the Nuremberg trials or the subsequent Code, it is noteworthy that its response to the injection project was an attempt to ensure that its contractor physicians agreed to certain standards in the use of human subjects. These standards were expressed in two 1947 letters, one in April and the other in November, from the AEC general manager in response to two different inquiries. The April letter required an "expectation that [research with human subjects] may have therapeutic effect," that official records can show that "each individual patient, being in an understanding state of mind, was clearly informed of the nature of the treatment and its possible effects, and expressed his willingness to receive the treatment." The letter also required that two physicians give written certification that these conditions have been satisfied (Wilson, 1947a). The November 1947 letter went still further, requiring that the "patient give his complete and informed consent in writing" (Wilson, 1947b).

In its capacity as an advisor to a subcommittee of the president's cabinet, and therefore indirectly advising the president himself, the ACHRE had to hew carefully to the evidence at hand. That evidence did not include specific reference to the Medical Trials, which were still taking place at Nuremberg in April 1947, or to the fact that they had been concluded by November of that year. The most that could be said with certainty was that the AEC was aware of the potentially harmful effect publicity about the plutonium injections could have, at least in legal and public relations terms, as evidenced by the March 1947 recommendation of its Medical Division and its Public Relations Department to continue the classified status of a paper about the experiment (Brundage, 1947). Similarly, an unsigned October 8, 1947, memorandum to the AEC's Advisory Board on Biology and Medicine suggested that "there is perhaps a greater responsibility if a federal agency condones human guinea pig experimentation" (Unknown author, 1947).

Yet it would have been remarkable if the lawyers and administrators who were charged with responsibility for the nation's nuclear arsenal and whose agency had virtually monopoly control over the availability or radioisotopes for medical or any other purposes had not taken note of the proceedings then taking place. The likelihood that they did is given further credence by a remark made by a high AEC official several years later, in 1950. The AEC and the Department of Defense (DOD) were engaged in planning a joint project called Nuclear Energy for the Propulsion of Aircraft (NEPA). A particular concern was the amount of radiation to which an air crew could safely be exposed by the energy source of the aircraft. One of the physician consultants was Robert Stone, who had been the recipient of the November 1947 letter from the AEC general manager that required "informed consent." Stone proposed that human experiments be performed as the only way of obtaining the needed information. But the chief of AEC's Division of Biology and Medicine, Shields Warren, objected. In a meeting of the AEC-DOD Joint Panel on the Medical Aspects of Atomic Warfare during which the use of "prisoner volunteers" was proposed, Warren replied: "It's not very long since we got through trying Germans for doing exactly the same thing" (Atomic Energy Commission, 1950b).

Furthermore, a 1951 exchange between the AEC's Division of Biology and Medicine and its Los Alamos Laboratory indicates that the spirit, if not the letter, of the Nuremberg Code was known outside the AEC's central office. A Los Alamos information officer, Leslie Redman, inquired about the AEC's policies on human experimentation, which were only vaguely known at the Lab (strongly suggesting that neither of the sets of rules in the two 1947 letters was widely disseminated). Redman said that his understanding was that "these regulations are comparable to those of the American Medical Association" (Redman, 1951). Thus, although Redman was not familiar with the two 1947 letters, the AMA principles did make an impression on the "culture" of radiation research, and we have seen that these were in essence the same as those expressed in the Nuremberg Code.

THE NUREMBERG CODE IN THE PENTAGON

The Joint Panel's proposal to conduct prisoner experiments that was opposed by the AEC's Shields Warren was also hotly debated in the Pentagon (all of these discussions were, of course, highly classified). Interestingly, the two major uniformed services, the navy and the army, split on the question in 1950, with the navy favoring the proposal and the army opposing it. The assistant secretary of the army argued that, instead, animal studies should be continued, and he noted that the Joint Panel's proposal had been rejected by the Committee on Medical Sciences of the Pentagon's Research and Development Board (Office of the Secretary of Defense, 1950). While the assistant secretary was technically correct, the Committee on Medical Sciences did not close off the possibility entirely, but referred the matter back to the Joint Panel for further consideration. At least two of the committee's physician members seemed to agree that such human studies could be done so long as they conformed with the December 1946 AMA principles (Department of Defense, 1950b). Clearly, by 1950 the AMA-Nuremberg principles were on the minds of many medical advisors in the national security establishment.

The human experimentation debate raged on in the Pentagon for the following two years. Finally, in mid-October 1952, a defense department lawyer named Stephen S. Jackson determined that the Nuremberg Code principles would have to be used in their entirety because they "already had international juridical sanction" (Rapalski, 1953). Jackson so advised the Armed Forces Medical Policy Council, a high-level Pentagon body that was chaired by Dr. Melvin Casberg. At their October 13, 1952, meeting the AFMPC recommended that the Department of Defense adopt the Nuremberg Code as its policy in the use of human experimental subjects, with one addition recommended by Jackson: that prisoners of war were explicitly ruled out as research participants (Rapalski, 1953).

The significance of Jackson's lawyerly conclusion should not be passed over lightly. It stands in remarkable contrast to the rejection of the Code by jurists decades later, when its principles were largely viewed as superseded by national security considerations, or even not recognized as in existence in the early 1950s (Annas, 1992). However, as the documentary evidence only recently available makes clear, in 1952 a Pentagon lawyer at least recognized Nuremberg as good law that applied to the United States Department of Defense. In this conclusion he was strongly supported by Assistant Secretary of Defense for Manpower and Personnel Anna M. Rosenberg. An expert on labor relations from New York, Rosenberg not only concurred in the Pentagon counsel's view but also recommended the addition of a clause that required the written consent of the potential subject (Jackson, 1952). Thus, in a memo dated January 13, 1953, the AFMPC wrote the secretary of defense that it "strongly recommended that a policy be established for the use of human volunteers (military and civilian employees) in experimental research at Armed Forces facilities," and that such use "shall be subject to the principles and conditions laid down as a result of the Nuremberg Trials" (Casberg, 1953).

But the path of the Nuremberg Code through the Pentagon hierarchy was still not a smooth one. Internal opposition to a written human subjects policy, or to any policy at all, was considerable; its "controversial character" was admitted by George V. Underwood, the director of the Executive Office of the Secretary of Defense early in January 1953 (Underwood, 1953a). Under-wood then attempted to win the strong endorsement of the proposal from the three uniformed service secretaries prior to the new administration of President-elect Eisenhower. This effort failed, and it was instead agreed that the matter should be called to the attention of Eisenhower's incoming secretary of defense, Charles E. Wilson, since he was the one who would have to implement it (Underwood, 1953b).

When the new secretary of defense approved the AFMPC's recommendation on February 26, 1953, he could not have had very much time to study what had perhaps been the single most debated subject in Pentagon medical circles for the previous three years. As the former chief executive of General Motors, Charles E. Wilson brought with him from the private sector an expeditious management style, one accustomed to relying on the judgment of responsible subordinates. No expert himself on medical issues, Wilson must have appreciated the need to prepare for expected Soviet and perhaps Red Chinese challenges in unconventional warfare. His experience in labor relations might also have taught him the importance of written contracts and protection from liability. The preamble to the Nuremberg Code–based memorandum specifies that the human experiments being contemplated are "the only feasible means for realistic evaluation and/or development of effective preventive measures of defense against atomic, biological or chemical agents" (Secretary of Defense, 1953).

THE NUREMBERG CODE MEETS
HARVARD MEDICAL SCHOOL

As several commentators have noted, the Nuremberg Code never established a firm foothold in statute or regulations in the United States. Partly this was due to the Code's failure to address research with those who were unable to give "voluntary consent," such as children, and partly to a cultural resistance to external regulation within the medical profession. In 1959 the National Society for Medical Research (NSMR) held a conference at the University of Chicago on legal issues in medicine. An NSMR Committee on the Re-Evaluation of the Nuremberg Experimental Principles recommended that consent be understood as "either explicit or reasonably presumed," and that third-parties be allowed to give permission for those who are incapable of consenting to research (*Report on the National Conference,* 1959).

From 1954 to 1964 the World Medical Association was engaged in a discussion of its own research code of ethics, often called the Helsinki Declaration. Developed by representatives of the medical research community itself, the Declaration differed from the Code in several important ways, including a more flexible view of subject consent when research participation can be considered to be potentially beneficial to the subject (World Medical Association, 1964). In 1961, several years before the Helsinki Declaration, administrators at Harvard Medical School became concerned about a new clause in its army medical research contracts, language that essentially reiterated the Nuremberg Code and applied it to the army's contract researchers as well as to research conducted by the army itself, as required by the 1953 Wilson memorandum. An assistant dean of the medical school, Dr. Joseph W. Gardella, wrote a memorandum in which he noted that "the Nuremberg Code was conceived in reference to Nazi atrocities. . . . The Code . . . is not necessarily pertinent to or adequate for the conduct of medical research in the United States" (1953). Gardella also questioned whether those who are sick are capable of understanding complex information, an issue that has been a concern of much of the more recent scholarship in biomedical ethics.

When Gardella presented his discussion to the medical school administrative board in 1962, a board member, Dr. Henry Beecher, agreed to draft a statement of Harvard's principles concerning human research. Beecher had already written on the subject of research ethics, and several years later he published a paper in the *New England Journal of Medicine* that contended there were numerous examples of the abuse of human subjects in the published medical literature. "Ethics and Clinical Research," which appeared in 1966, proved to be one of the most influential events in the history of modern medical ethics. However, Beecher relied less on subject consent as a protection for research participants, particularly those who are ill, than he did on the relationship between the patient and his or her physician. In short order, Beecher and his

Harvard colleagues succeeded in persuading the army to permit them to substitute their principles for the Nuremberg Code language in their research contracts (ACHRE, 1996).

CHANGING A PROFESSIONAL CULTURE

The failure of the AEC and the Pentagon policies to penetrate the cultures of their respective professional communities provides an important lesson about the reform of deeply ingrained practices among highly trained experts. In both cases, lawyers and nonphysician administrators attempted to impose conditions that were regarded as irrelevant or unrealistic by medical researchers. Although there was apparently willingness to accept AEC central office research requirements at the contract laboratories, it is important to appreciate that by the early 1950s the human subjects exposed to ionizing radiation for experimental purposes were mainly normal volunteers. By contrast, in the late 1940s those who were subjects in radiation experiments were often sick patients for whom the appropriateness of a consent process was met with much skepticism. We saw the same dynamic at work fifteen years later in the NSMR committee report, in Harvard Medical School's reception of the Nuremberg Code clause in its army contracts, and in the Helsinki Declaration itself.

To appreciate the true influence of the Code, one must abandon the expectation that, to be influential, it would have to be immediately and openly accepted and integrated into the actual practices of the research community. Instead, the Code's attempt to articulate the ethics of research was flawed, and the initial reception given it by most researchers was also flawed. Nevertheless, the root principle of consent proved hard to ignore. Even as efforts were made to massage and transform it, events such as the thalidomide tragedy and the Tuskegee study in the 1960s and 1970s brought home its forceful truth, however poorly expressed. With a logic that seems inexorable in retrospect, the Code was first seen as obviously applying to imprisoned and oppressed persons, then to all healthy subjects, then to those who were sick but would not benefit from an experiment, and finally to those who were sick but stood a chance of benefiting from research participation. In fact, it was not logic that was operative in this evolution, but a growth in moral perception.

Although the principle of informed consent to research participation is now well established, even for those who are sick, there is still reluctance among many medical professionals to accept that patients facing serious medical problems are able to process information about innovative therapies. The ACHRE's Subject Interview Study of hundreds of patients throughout the country found varying levels of understanding of research but widespread trust among research subjects in medical professionals and medical institutions (ACHRE, 1996). The juxtaposition of limited understanding and exceptional trust gives reason for concern about the consequences if the public begins to discern reasons to be more skeptical of the research enterprise.

NOTE

The author worked on the staff of the Advisory Committee on Human Radiation Experiments. The views expressed in the two papers in this section are those of the author and do not represent the views of the Advisory Committee. The findings, recommendations, and analysis of the Advisory Committee are expressed in the "Final Report of the Advisory Committee on Human Radiation Experiments," available from Oxford University Press under the title *The Human Radiation Experiments* (New York, 1996).

Most of the material used in this chapter and the previous one is also analyzed in Part One of the Advisory Committee's final report, most of which I was responsible for organizing and drafting. However, the final report was the product of the work of many talented scholars and scientists, and I gratefully acknowledge their influence on my understanding of this material.

PART FIVE
NEW DIRECTIONS

Introduction

Even those of us who have the luxury of following bioethics issues for a living seem to find it ever more difficult to stay on top of the relevant scientific developments and commentary on their ethical and social implications. Sometime in the early 1990s the idea that one could be a bioethical generalist became less plausible. People started concentrating on clinical ethics, research ethics, ethics and genetics, public health ethics, and others that I would mention if the field could agree on the categories.

This section considers various novel challenges to bioethics, challenges that have appeared in different forms. One chapter is also frankly personal: the intersection of my mother's serious medical problem when she was not yet 40, my own fortieth birthday, and the moral and epistemological puzzles associated with genetics and clinical medicine.

The chapter on "neuroethics" came at the invitation of *Nature Reviews Neuroscience* after I participated in a Dana Foundation workshop on this emerging area, but the greatly enhanced technology for investigating the living brain and nervous system have been sneaking up on us for some time, making possible a level of understanding that was out of reach when brain research was limited mostly to animals or to human cadavers. In contrast to all the ink that has been spilled on ethics and genetics, neuroscience has been relatively neglected by writers in bioethics.

Less than two weeks after September 11, 2001, I sat with my laptop in a nearly empty Buffalo, New York, airport waiting for one of the few flights to Washington, D.C., available and contemplating the implications of recent events for various bioethical issues. I have received more reactions to "Bioethics after the Terror" than to any other short piece I have ever written.

I conclude with reflections on some of the problems confronting bioethics as a profession. Bioethics is well into its fourth decade as a self-conscious area of study (at least in the United States). It is time this post-adolescent accepted that external scrutiny is needed now, and that the need won't go away.

12

Cancer, Truth, and Genetics

TRUTH AND CONSEQUENCES

When I turned 40, I experienced the usual twinge associated with full awareness that mortality was no longer a theoretical possibility, even if I never got hit by a car. I also had another experience, one shared by many with certain family health histories. When I was five years old and my mother was just shy of her fortieth birthday, she was diagnosed with a chondrosarcoma in her upper arm.

The problem took a year to diagnose in those days, the mid-1950s. My father, a physician, sought advice from colleagues in several states and in Europe. By the time the condition was finally accurately diagnosed (after numerous theories, from arthritis to hysteria had been rejected), the tumor had assumed the size of an egg-shaped lump and my mother was in constant pain. When radical amputation including the shoulder was recommended (perhaps limb-sparing surgery would have been considered today), she was actually relieved. At least that pain would stop.

This story had a happy ending. As I write, my mother is still alive. Now 87 years old, she has enjoyed a career as an internationally recognized psychotherapist. Her subsequent health was quite stable until the infirmities of old age caught up with her, but even now she is very resilient.

One aspect of her experience continues to annoy her though. A few years after her amputation, she was looking for something in my father's desk drawer when she found a letter from her surgeon to my father. The letter indicated that her prognosis was excellent if she survived the first five years post-amputation. This is a conversation that none of her physicians ever had with her, only with her physician husband.

I tell this story whenever I teach my first-year medical students about truth-telling. The approach my mother's surgeon took was quite conventional at that time. A 1961 survey reported that about 90 percent of physicians said they rarely or never used the word *cancer* with their patients, preferring to employ euphemisms like "growth" (Oken 1961). Less than twenty years later a similar survey (Novack et al., 1979) found exactly the opposite result: Around 90 percent of the physicians said they always or usually used the word *cancer.*

Clearly, many factors combined to change attitudes in the ensuing twenty years, including much better cancer therapies and vastly altered popular feeling about self-determination, that is, that people have the right to know the truth about their medical condition. Today we take this view for granted, and it is startling to consider how much matters have changed in so little time.

This conversion, while generally good for patients who want control over their lives and their medical decision making, has undoubtedly made it more challenging for their doctors. They must navigate between a desire to protect people from devastating personal news (which no one enjoys delivering), and the obligation to tell people the truth.

More problematic still is the fact that the "truth" about one's medical condition has become a much more complex matter than it was half a century ago, especially in light of probabilistic genetics. The odd feeling I experienced when I passed my mother's age with no cancer diagnosis, even knowing that there was no reason to believe I was at significant increased risk, made me wonder what I would do if there were a way to calculate my chances.

Would I want to know? At what age would I want to know? How would the information affect my life? And what is "knowledge" when we are talking about probabilities? At some point risks can be so remote that to say one "knows" them has little meaning. If I know that I have a one in a million chance of being struck by lightning, what do I really know?

THE INFORMATION ILLUSION

The human desire for knowledge must be closely tied to our evolutionary history and to the importance of knowledge for survival through control of our immediate environment. Perhaps that is why we are flummoxed by information that is breathtakingly precise but largely useless, even damaging. This is the point behind the distinction so often made today between information and knowledge. For example, Web surfers in search of medical information can be flooded with detail that lacks context and perspective and is therefore often worse than having no information at all.

Even risks that involve very high probabilities but about which we can do little convey more information than they do knowledge. One of the surprises about early screening programs for Huntington's disease was how few people at risk decided to find out whether they had a 50 percent chance of getting the disease. Only around a third of them decided to be tested. Early bioethicists coined the term "genetic prophecy" to describe information that enabled little if any control over the future events described.

In oncology, genetic screening for breast cancer has received the most attention in ethics literature and in public discussion. As is so often the case, a unique combination of events has driven this interest: a scientific achievement (the identification of markers), a technological breakthrough (the development of an assay), and a disease associated with great suffering and with parts of the human body that are fraught with powerful symbolism (organs related to reproduction).

It also happened to be the case that a group in which the relevant genetic alterations appear to be prevalent, Ashkenazi Jews, was willing to participate in the early trials. Considering that I am a medical school professor, I learned about these studies from an unlikely source, when my son's backpack included a flyer from his Jewish day school announcing that subjects were being sought. There was no trouble enrolling subjects, at least in the early studies, because the Jewish community was eager to participate. Concerns grew, however, when the prevalence of BRCA1/2 alterations became more widely known. Anti-Semitic Web sites began to reference these results as evidence of racial inferiority. Science advisory groups were in this way reminded that genetic studies carry with them a risk of group stigmatization, a problem that is now widely recognized and is supposed to be assessed when research protection programs review proposals involving the genomes of certain groups.

Similarly, some anxiety has greeted the National Institutes of Health's "HapMap" project, which is an attempt to determine how the inheritance of large blocks of genes is related to disease patterns in populations. Such concerns should not, of course, put a stop to science, but they do signal the sensitivity attached to genetic issues and the need to respond. Fortunately the NIH seems to be acutely aware of this problem. There is also an important lesson in the exaggerated significance the public associates with genes, and that points to a long-term educational effort that doctors and scientists need to undertake. The scientific world's appropriate excitement about genetics has created a popular conception of genetic reductionism. Many people seem to think that everything about us in "in our genes" and fail to appreciate that our DNA generally is but one factor among many in determining our characteristics and our destiny.

APPROACH WITH CAUTION

All of this brings me back to my forty-ish twinge regarding my own genetic status. Ten years ago the American Society for Human Genetics (ASHG) published guidelines for BRCA1 testing that still incorporate some important and generalizable principles:[1]

First, testing should be "direct and reliable"; that is, the science and the technology should be at a point that justifies clinical use.

---

1. http://genetics.faseb.org/genetics/ashg/pubs/policy/pol-11.htm

At that point it might be offered to individuals with strong family histories, but until then it should only be investigational. Substantial self-discipline is required of the medical profession to adhere to such a condition, and unfortunately that has not always characterized the introduction of new treatment approaches.

Second, it will still be important, before the testing comes into wide use, for the best monitoring and prevention strategies to be identified. The subsequent experience with bone marrow transplantation for breast cancer is eloquent testimony to the importance of sound trials before an implicit (and perhaps unjustified) standard of care is realized. As exciting as high-tech interventions can be, and as much as they might appeal to our intuitions about likely success, they are often not the most effective ones and might even do more harm than good.

Third, population-based screening should be approached warily. Probability of occurrence, efficacy, and safety of follow-up must all be well understood before such measures are considered. Inaccurate predictions could be devastating. Population-based screening that is not sensitively managed can also lead to group stigmatization and subsequent mistrust that backfires, as in the case of sickle cell screening for African-Americans in the early 1970s.

Finally, as I have mentioned, public education is crucial. In this respect, the stakes are even higher now that one company has taken the first steps toward direct-to-consumer promotion of a home-based breast cancer genetic test. When I was interviewed on this subject by the *Boston Globe* in the spring of 2003, following the announcement of the company's intentions, I expressed concern that public understanding simply isn't sufficient to justify such marketing. Consumers who are interested in home testing should first be asked to agree to participate in a monitored educational program, preferably in concert with their personal physician. If ever the ancient Hippocratic maxim "First do no harm" applied to something, it applies here. I gather that, in this case, the company has decided to continue to engage the patient's physician in the decision whether to test.

This last point goes to the market-driven nature of so much modern medicine. This is perhaps the most important element of the real-world consequences of ever more sophisticated genetic medicine. I am not a pessimist in this regard because I believe that if the medical profession adopts a strong position, doctors can avoid becoming dispensers of genetic tests upon demand. As the technology becomes more inviting for self-determining consumers, the need for professional judgment will only increase.

13

Neuroethics:
An Agenda for Neuroscience and Society

Announcing the arrival of neuroethics, the Charles W. Dana Foundation at Stanford University sponsored a highly publicized conference on May 13–14, 2002, in San Francisco, in which I participated. The multidisciplinary sessions included talks by leading scientists on various aspects of neuroscience with reactions from philosophers, law professors, bioethicists, and science educators.

Some participants wondered about an analogy with the 1975 Asilomar conference on the potential hazards of recombinant DNA technology. Unlike Asilomar, however, there is currently no widespread public clamor for self-restraint on the part of the relevant scientific community. If anything, there is a broad-based fascination with the prospects of neuroscience-based innovation, especially as awareness of the ravages of neurological diseases has grown and as aging baby boomers hope that science will help them extend their own mental acuity. Early rDNA technology was not nearly as steeped in commercial opportunities as is current neuroscience, which operates amid the lucrative environment created by modern psychopharmacology.

FREE WILL AND MIND-BODY REDUCTIONISM

Yet there are longstanding issues concerning the control or alteration of mind and brain that are sure to surface again. There is no better example than that of free will and determinism, a potential philosophical quagmire that has, since the ancient Greeks, inspired some of the most imaginative intellectual footwork. Does our growing knowledge about the origins and physical basis of mental states, let alone the possibility of controlling them with some specificity, further threaten liberal ideals of freedom and personal responsibility? In short, is neuroscience on the road to demonstrating, once and for all, that mental states reduce to brain states, and even to brain states that may be subject to direct manipulation?

Consider the following results that exemplify what some may find disturbing about information provided by the new brain science. Drawing on event-related fMRI data, investigators found that social judgments about trustworthiness appear to be based on facial representations involving the extrastriate visual cortices in the fusiform and superior temporal gyri. Perceptual processing is then linked to social judgments drawing on the amygdala and regions of the prefrontal and somatosensory cortices (Winston et al., 2002). Similarly, Stanford researchers have developed evidence that the fusiform region is involved in the preferential response to faces of one's own race (Golby et al., 2001). What implications do such data have for the notion of free will?

There are several different concerns here that should not be conflated:

1. Is the mental reducible to the physical?

2. If the mental is reducible to the physical, does that imply that there is no freedom of the will?

3. If the mental can be controlled by physical manipulation, does that imply that there is no freedom of the will?

Even if 1 is true, it does not follow that free will is an illusion, nor does it follow that cases in which the mental is manipulated cannot be distinguished from cases in which it is not, though the challenges involved in drawing such distinctions may be formidable.

Begin with the problem of mind-body reductionism, one that is vexed with imprecise language, including the notion of reduction itself. Probably the most widely admired contemporary treatment of this and related issues is that of Patricia Churchland. Well before the current enthusiasm for neuroethics, Churchland published her landmark *Neurophilosophy* (1989). Churchland canvassed the various meanings of reduction and traced the epistemological debates behind them, noting that the underlying question is which theory of the mind is reducible to which theory of the brain, or vice versa. There is, as she points out, no received view of the interconnections between mental states and behavior, but upon analysis, the notion that there could be such a theory is neither implausible nor necessarily offensive. As I shall note shortly, philosophers have been living with this possibility for a long time while managing to preserve useful ideas like freedom of the will.

The view that there is something offensive about intertheoretic reduction appears to rest on the notion that there is something inherently objectionable about the idea that nonphysical brain states can be explained in terms of neuronal states. Dualists and non-dualists have raised such objections, but they do not seem persuasive. For example, the view that the mental and the physical are two distinct substances has a hard time explaining their interaction, as in evolution.

A more subtle position has it that mental properties are distinct from physical properties, so that mental experience may at most be said to emerge from the physical. Here a great burden is placed on the notion of emergence, which appears to rule out a comprehensive neurobiological theory. Yet various difficulties infect emergentist views, including that in at least some cases they run aground on the intentional fallacy, in which thoughts about objects are mistaken for properties of the objects themselves. Still another set of objections to intertheoretic reduction argue that the logic of nonphysical description is distinct from the logic of physical description, that the relations between the sentences used to describe one domain are different from those used to describe another. Here again, the appeal is to folk psychology. But if not all cognitive activity operates like language (as is the case for some models of information storage or seemingly intelligent animal communication), then sentential relations need not be the ultimate appeal, and it remains an empirical question whether folk psychology may not be improved to the point of radical transformation by neuroscientific insights.

Meanwhile, we are left with a more-or-less serviceable theory of the mental that Churchland calls "folk psychology," the commonsense means at our disposal to explain behavior with reference to beliefs, desires, expectations, goals, and so on. Scientific discoveries in the neurosciences (proceeding perhaps from the kinds of examples I will consider shortly), may require gradual improvements in folk psychology. These improvements, she observes, may proceed so gradually that folk psychology will come to be seen as having been replaced rather than reduced to a theory of the brain.

Suppose that, as seems likely, the reductionist debate continues indefinitely. As the hypothesized ongoing refinement of folk psychology by improved neuroscientific understanding takes place, history gives reason to believe that the idea of free will may be left standing. To the fledgling student, the issue of freedom and causation has long seemed an enticing and hopeless quandary, the Scylla and Charybdis of psychology. But the most notable thinkers have been unruffled by the matter, often taking a middle-ground position known as "soft determinism," the view that we are capable of entering into the chain of causes of our thoughts and actions. That is, although my individual psychology and experience shape my preferences, they do not do so in detail, and I am capable of inserting more or less original choices into the chain of causes. Thus, even knowing the whole of a person's reinforcement history would not be sufficient to predict all their behaviors. Recent analytic philosophers have gone so far as to call free will and determinism a pseudo-problem, one that subsists only in the linguistic expressions available to us.

It is worth recalling in an overview like this one that the most important precursor of modern neuroscience was William James, the Harvard-trained physician who spent much of his career reflecting on the implications of psychology for philosophy. James's typically vigorous take on the question of free will was to assert what he called "the will to believe," that is, that the fact of free will could be established by the act of determining to believe in it. What refutation to such a declaration is possible? If either option is equally plausible, he argued, one might as well reach for the more attractive of the two. James's approach is perhaps more compelling in the context of his remarkable *Principles of Psychology,* published in 1890, in which he elaborated virtually all of what was then known about the brain and nervous system into a coherent psychological theory.

Of particular importance for James were the implications of this information for moral development. In this respect he followed a long line from Aristotle and helped the philosopher John Dewey develop his influential theory of education in which the development of sound learning habits is viewed as more important than absorbing factual content. The original soft determinist, Aristotle argued that individuals are partly responsible for the kind of person they become, for example, by choosing those with whom they associate, which in turn influences their own moral character. James continued a tradition that Aristotle started in the analysis of habit formation. He applied the early lessons of neurophysiology to admonitions about launching strongly and repeatedly on any new behavior in order to establish a pattern in neural material that will increase the likelihood that the behavior will be repeated, and gradually with less effort. Within a few years, Dewey designed a school intended to bolster habits of inquisitiveness and problem-solving skills, the beginning of the progressive education movement.

All this is by way of pointing out that the ground has long been prepared for anticipated transformations in folk psychology by previous generations of thinkers who observed such changes in their own lifetimes and seem to have expected them to continue. This is not to say that the process has been or will be without stress, both at the level of theory and at the level of social practices. In the rest of this survey, I will allude to examples of these stress points and their implications, proceeding roughly from the more immediate to the science fictional. However far-fetched, the latter are appropriate areas for the ethics of neuroscience. The point of such a discourse is not merely to assess the implications of brain science for topics of more immediate concern, such as changing ideas about legal responsibility, but also to consider the social consequences over the longer term.

REDUCTIONISM *REDUX*

The legal system is of course at the frontier of formal social responses to advances in scientific understanding of human behavior. Numerous courts have already begun to assess defense strategies involving medications that were alleged to compromise the defendants' *mens rea*, the state of mind required for culpability. A number of such cases have involved individuals who were undergoing treatment with fluoxetine (marketed under the trade name Prozac). In these cases, the courts have focused on expert testimony concerning the causal role of the medication in the commission of a crime (2002 WL 31553982 [Ga. App.]).

As the legal system is inclined to look to the scientific community for guidance in establishing culpability when psychoactive medication is implicated (thus playing an important role in the modification of folk psychology), it will also do so in cases of traumatic brain injury. Such cases involving the prefrontal region have been observed as leaving the patient with adequate moral reasoning but without the capacity to act upon an appropriate conclusion. Improved imaging and diagnostic techniques, particularly if damage to the ventromedial sector can be identified, show promise for identifying similar cases that stem from nontraumatic disorders. Thus a more nuanced approach to offenders whose behavior can be correlated with trauma in certain neurologic systems seems inevitable.

A reasoned respect for the law depends in part on the extent to which findings of culpability are consistent with the best available evidence about self-determination. As Damasio (1994) notes, a criminal who is evidently brain damaged has the moral status of a patient whose condition could properly be brought under a medical rubric. But emerging data suggest that the traditional category of "criminal insanity" may not necessarily apply to an individual who is capable of *understanding* but not *appreciating* the difference between right and wrong; where (to use Damasio's terms), understanding is a function of the reasoning/decision making system and appreciation is a function of the emotion/feeling system. It seems inevitable that further categories will have to be developed to capture more precise senses of culpability, as has already begun in cases involving psychoactive drugs.

A far different and more speculative sort of problem with the law arises from the possibility that individuals may be able to deliberately forget actions for which they should be held culpable but for which the evidence is circumstantial. Work by M. C. Anderson suggests that individuals who have been abused by parents are able to intentionally repress those memories (Levy and Anderson, 2002). Clearly, in these cases there is a powerful psychological impetus to forget trauma at the hands of those upon whom one is dependent. It would be interesting to know if the same mechanism can be used to forget selected events or actions even without the same emotional drive, and if physiological indicators like galvanic skin response can also be inhibited. Psychologically sophisticated offenders would thus be handed a new tool to evade prosecution.

PERSONAL IDENTITY

Closely related to issues about free will are concerns about personal identity. The last few years have already witnessed a vigorous debate about the implications of fluoxetine (Prozac) and other selective serotonin reuptake inhibitors. These psychopharmacologic interventions appear to be longer lasting and perhaps more pervasive in their effects on the human personality than more familiar mind-altering substances, with fewer unwanted effects. However, the ethical issues raised in connection with the newer psychoactive drugs may not be different in kind from assertions that these or any other alterations of mentation or conduct are "artificial" and therefore suspect. To make such assertions stick, a background theory of the "natural" is required, a challenging job in itself. In any case, the decision to use a drug that modifies one's personality may be a free choice, at least in the sense of soft determinism, and therefore an expression of authentic personality.

So long as the effects of medications end as they leave the system, there can be a return to baseline and individual choice about continuing or not. A more ethically challenging scenario runs as follows: Suppose we have the ability to permanently alter the brain stem or basal forebrain nuclei that deliver serotonin, among other neurotransmitters. In primates, it has been found that the greater number of serotonin-2 receptors, the less aggressive and more social the behavior. Suppose, further, that neuronal deficiency can be determined in at least some extremely hostile individuals. For those who have trouble controlling their hostile behavior, drug therapy would no longer be needed if the number of crucial neurons were increased to the normal range. Old-fashioned psychosurgery, classically in the form of a prefrontal lobotomy, deforms normal structure. Would this newer form of psychosurgery be acceptable if were seen as helping the brain attain the physiologic standard?

New brain tissue grafts are only one sort of medical intervention suggested by information about the relationship between neurons and behavior. Another study leads to the intersection of neuroscience with genetics and prenatal diagnosis. University of Wisconsin investigators reported that members of a group of men who were both abused as children and had an alteration in the gene responsible for producing monoamine oxidase A (MAOA), were nine times as likely to commit criminal or antisocial acts as normal controls (Caspi et al., 2002). If this or other neurotransmitters come to be roughly associated with socially offensive behavior even under less extreme environmental insults, they could be brought within the controversy over preimplantation genetic diagnosis. Prospective parents might thus submit embryos to testing for the MAOA marker prior to implantation in order to avoid giving birth to a child with this particular potential for criminality.

A more general approach to disorders of brain development is being pursued by a Harvard and Beth Israel (Boston) Medical Center team. This group reports that it has already identified some of the genetic alterations that result in brains that are too small, abnormally patterned, or evidence abnormal location of cortical cells. Specifically, they report that the cerebral cortex of transgenic mice with an alteration in the B-catenin exhibited formations of gyri and sulci, which are found in the brains of lower animals.

The Boston group theorizes that B-catenin regulated the proliferation of progenitor cells that lead to a thickened cortical sheet, as found in human beings (Chenn and Walsh, 2002).

Although it is, of course, far too early to assess the relation of the B-catenin regulator to intelligence, results like these may lead us to think about developing diagnostic tests for disorders such as mental retardation or epilepsy. Suppose that this kind of work eventually leads to the management of at least some of the mechanisms that control the functional performance of the brain. One can only imagine the pressure to bring to fruition one of the great science fiction scenarios: genetic engineering that not only corrects for the presence of genes that code for conditions recognized as obvious disorders but actually seeks to enhance mental capacity.

Examples like this suggest that neuroethical debates are unlikely to appear wholly separate from more familiar bioethical issues that arise in genetics and reproduction. An example of a controversy that, in retrospect, could be brought under the ambit of neuroethics was the use of fetal tissue for implantation in the brains of sufferers from Parkinson's and other neurological diseases. In the late 1980s claims of success made by surgeons in Mexico and Sweden stimulated a debate about the acceptability of using fetal brain tissue in this way. Unfortunately, the early hopes for the procedure have not in any case been realized, but the incident foreshadowed the current dispute about embryonic stem cells.

IMPAIRED CONSENT

To this list of previous neuroethics issues one may add experiments with persons whose decision-making capacity, and hence their ability to give valid consent, is impaired. This is a surprisingly old problem, with governments in Europe and the United States trying to set policies as long ago as 1900. Institutionalized persons, including the mentally ill, have long been favorite research subjects because they are confined and can be monitored. Historically, experiments involving asylum inmates have not always been confined to conditions from which they suffered. Often they were "animals of necessity" for experiments that required human models. Gradually, law, policy, and public outcry have made persons with mental disorders less desirable subjects (Moreno, 1998).

The opportunity to diagnose and treat dementing maladies, a cutting edge led by research on Alzheimer's disease, has led to renewed attention to the ethics of research with impaired or absent decision-making ability. Imaging techniques, sometimes combined with agents intended to provoke neurological processes, have created enormous pressures on the old consensus. Some agreement has crystallized around the proposition that it is possible to devise protections for those with decisional impairments that are consistent with low-risk experimental procedures or those that, while of higher risk, carry some potential benefit to the patient. However, stumbling blocks remain. One is the uncertainty about who may authorize such research if the patient cannot, an especially serious issue for incapacitated adults. Many of the lessons that may be learned from basic research with impaired brains, as well as innovative translations of neuroscientific discoveries to clinical medicine, turn on the social question of who may give permission on behalf of those who cannot give it themselves (National Bioethics Advisory Commission, 1999).

A different sort of quandary sits on the border between research and therapy. Early detection of lesions associated with Alzheimer's will perhaps be only the leading edge of diagnostic tools for neurologic disorders in the preclinical state, disorders for which there are no effective therapies. In this sort of case, the capacity of the patient at the time of testing is not in doubt. A number of those at risk for Alzheimer's may request brain imaging. Some clinicians will view testing for risk status as appropriate, arguing that it will facilitate long-term planning; others will urge that any such detection should only take place as part of a clinical trial until a medical intervention is available. Some consensus will be required concerning appropriate counseling in such cases.

In instances such as this, one may learn from history. When pre-symptomatic diagnosis for Huntington's disease became available, some expected a rush to testing. But in the absence of an adequate intervention, many have opted against knowing their genetically determined destiny. If ignorance is not exactly bliss, neither is knowledge power in the absence of an implementing technique.

MANIPULATIONS, NATURAL AND NOT

Some neuroscientific discoveries, once they become more widely appreciated, are likely to become objects of popular imagination. Magnetic resonance imaging (MRI) studies conducted by colleagues at Emory University indicate that women who undertook cooperative acts during Prisoner's Dilemma Game trials experienced activation of dopamine-rich neurons (Rilling et al., 2002). Businesses valuing socially cooperative employees might be interested in such measures of the proclivities of prospective workers as a hiring screen, even though they may add nothing to psychological testing and letters of reference from previous employers. On the other hand, firms interested in more competitive types might use a pre-employment MRI to ferret out those who experience less pleasure from cooperation. It would be interesting to know whether these scans will be received as unacceptably invasive or just part of the job search routine.

A different sort of competitive advantage may be sought by ardent lovers with just enough neuroscientific knowledge to be dangerous. Investigators recently reported that thin, slow cortical fibers are associated with the pleasure that comes from a loving touch. These fibers connect to the somatosensory system and are present at birth, while the thicker fibers that rapidly convey sensation develop somewhat later. The Swedish and Canadian team theorizes that the infant is therefore capable of experiencing the emotional effect of parental touching before the tactile sensation itself (Olaussen et al., 2002). Considering the profound psychological depth of these feelings, unscrupulous lotharios may someday find techniques for thin fiber stimulation to be critical parts of their arsenal.

Aristotle's taxonomic biology, built around the classification of flora and fauna into genus and species, helped give credence to his metaphysical doctrine of natural kinds. Ever since, the notion of species mixing has been taken as "unnatural." Natural law philosophy draws moral implications from this doctrine, with bestiality as a prime example of a crime against nature based on the essential distinctness of natural kinds. When a presidential commission on ethics set out early rules for genetic engineering in the 1980s, the "species barrier" was cited as one to be respected.

To paraphrase Justice O'Connor's famous remark on the trimester scheme for regulation of abortion, the species barrier is a standard at war with itself. A pincer movement has been established by the results of comparative genome projects on one side and the need for animal models with telescoped life spans for critical medical research on the other. Both undermine commitment to the view that each species has its own unique essence.

Studies that aim to produce genetically altered rodents with human neurons are an interesting example and may someday test public tolerance of species mixing. Researchers have identified one among presumably very many genes linked to human speech. But this particular gene, FOXP2, is especially important because it appears to have conferred tremendous evolutionary advantage around 200,000 years ago when modern humans appeared (Editorial, 2002). To test this claim, the creation of a genetically modified mouse with the FOXP2 alteration seems the obvious next step. Interesting changes in physiology and behavior would presumably not include a talking mouse, as one of the investigators joked to the media, but at what point if any would the public find the presence of human neural tissue in mice to be an intolerable breach of the species barrier? It may only be fortuitous that the creation of mice that are transgenic for the Huntington's disease gene has not already aroused public anxiety about species mixing.

Once again, there are historic analogies to be drawn. Initial discomfort with porcine heart valves and other animal-to-human tissue grafts have given way to routine, in spite of continuing concern about the introduction of animal viruses into humans. Neural tissue, however, may push up against what Leon Kass, chairman of the president's Council on Bioethics calls "the wisdom of repugnance," especially if more than a tiny proportion of neurons is involved. A mouse with a brain entirely constructed from human neurons would surely provide remarkable research opportunities as well as likely prompting a national debate.

MIND WARS

During the 1940s and 1950s, the bulk of psychological research funding was provided by national security agencies interested in gaining an advantage during the cold war. Many of the scandals associated with this research, such as the CIA and army experiments with LSD and other hallucinogens, have become part of our cultural legacy (Moreno, 1999). They have also spawned a legion of conspiracy theorists prepared to entertain any rumored "mind-control" technology without being inhibited by scientific implausibility. Nonetheless, national security agencies continue to be interested in the benefits that could be conferred by scientific breakthroughs, as is demonstrated by the U.S. government's current attempt to control the publication of data deemed related to national security that has been obtained through research supported by federal grants or contracts. Paranoia and naiveté about these matters are not the only alternatives.

One favorite worry of conspiracy theorists is of that of long-range surveillance by state authorities. The introduction of increasingly sophisticated imaging technologies, such as fMRI is likely to give such fears a field day. Perhaps these fears would not be without merit. If devices based on these principles could be small and sensitive enough to detect high blood flow in neural systems associated with violence, they would be of great interest for use in airports and other sensitive public spaces. Individuals who trip these alarms could be stopped and interviewed or simply closely monitored while in the facility through the already ubiquitous video surveillance system. The civil liberties issues at stake here hardly require elaboration.

The potential military applications of neuroscientific developments are rarely mentioned in the literature. An exception is Daniel L. Schacter, who in *The Seven Sins of Memory* gives an example related to the gene that codes for the *N*-methyl-D-aspartate (NMDA) receptor. As it is linked to synaptic plasticity, mice with extra copies of NMDA demonstrated superior learning skills. Schacter notes that, if NMDA proves to have the memory-improving properties the early work indicates, it may not only lead to a useful therapy for people with memory disorders, but it may also be useful in those with normal memories. Again we approach the question of whether such genetic intervention in brain processes is acceptable and under what conditions (Schacter, 2001).

Particularly striking is Schacter's report of an observation by neurobiologist Tim Tully. A pacifist, Tully acknowledges that memory-enhancing medications would be very attractive in the heat of combat, when complex information about, say, a target-rich bombing mission must be apprehended by fighter pilots in a short time and many details stored. Schacter's allusion to the national security angle of the fruits of neuroscience, brief as it is, is nonetheless one of the few such references one sees in this literature.

One need not, of course, adopt Tully's view of the matter. As is the case for researchers in other fields, the post-9/11 environment should prompt a discussion about the moral responsibilities of neuroscientists that includes the aims and implications of their work, with particular attention to the agendas of various funding sources. In other words, they will need to join the ranks of atomic physicists and geneticists in shouldering a moral crucible. If the neurosciences are indeed poised for their own great leap forward, such will be the burdens of success.

IS NEUROETHICS NEW?

The frequent references made in this paper both to major historic figures in philosophy and science, and to issues and debates of longstanding have perhaps tipped the reader to my view that neuroethics is in some ways old wine in a new bottle. There is no reason for surprise here, and some reason for comfort. Ethical problems seem never to be wholly new; there are always precursors and therefore analogies to be drawn and prior conceptual schemes to be considered and revised or reformed. To the extent that there is an appearance of novelty as ethical issues come to widespread awareness, it is mainly because of peculiar aspects of a particular case that oblige a novel analytic approach. In the early days of bioethics, many issues attracted attention because of new technological capabilities such as the implications of life-extending modalities for the definition of clinical death. With its access to improving technologies, especially functional imaging, work now proceeding in the neurosciences provides rich ground for such cases. Many of those engaged in these efforts will find themselves the subjects of the sort of public attention previously experienced by their colleagues in nuclear physics and genetics. Neuroscientists will increasingly be challenged to explain the significance of their work in moral as well as scientific terms.

14

Bioethics after the Terror

There is no more trivial yet fundamental observation about bioethics than that it is a child of the 1960s. Not only the civil rights movements but also a generalized skepticism about establishment institutions nourished a field that made the reevaluation of medical paternalism and the establishment of patient self-determination central to a critique of physician-patient relations, a critique unprecedented in its scope and eventual success. Like so much of the sensibility of the 1960s, bioethics itself has become part of the establishment, as have those who profess it.

It should not be surprising, therefore, if certain themes that are characteristic of bioethics should be caught up in historic shifts in cultural sensibilities. What if individual autonomy and patient self-determination were no longer self-evident primary values in our public discourse? What if efficiency concerns about resource allocation were thought more respectable as compared to individual access to health care than has generally been the case? What if the public and the courts were less sympathetic to claims from persons who believe themselves to have been victimized by careless or unscrupulous experimenters for the sake of the greater good, particularly if those experiments had a national security purpose?

It is too early to tell if the tragic events of September 11, 2001, presage a significant or enduring cultural shift in American attitudes toward the way personal self-determination is factored into our civic life. Much will of course depend on the outcome of the current international crisis as well as its longevity. In the meantime, it is well to reflect on the favorable relationship mainstream bioethical constructs have enjoyed with mainstream cultural values. Up to now, bioethics and those who espouse the study of moral values in the life sciences have been on the right side of history, for that history has been characterized by intensifying concern about human rights. As a result, bioethicists have been privileged to participate in a social agenda that has won widespread approbation, first in public media and finally even in the healthcare institutions that once resisted these "strangers at the bedside," in David Rothman's felicitous phrase (1991).

Here I examine some potential implications for bioethics—understood as a body of moral theory as well as a set of social practices—that could create novel tensions for a field that has never experienced a fundamental shift in the priorities of its surrounding culture. Only one assumption need be made for this analysis to proceed: that no intellectual pursuit that keeps at least one eye fixed on public affairs can remain apart from the sort of sea change that we might now be witnessing.

ALL-TOO-HUMAN EXPERIMENTS

One week before the attacks on the World Trade Center and the Pentagon, the U.S. government admitted that it had developed a version of an anthrax strain believed to be held in Russian stockpiles. No contravention of the treaty permitting only defensive bioweapons research was admitted, for these projects were aimed at *preventing* a successful attack and government officials reasoned that research aimed at defense could only be effective if undertaken in light of the potentialties of actual offensive devices (*Washington Post*, 5 September 2001).

I confess to having been somewhat taken aback by this revelation, not, I hope, out of any naiveté about the need for continued biodefense work or by the thin line between defensive and offensive research. Rather, I recalled the many questions I received while promoting a book on the history and ethics of national security experiments, when both sophisticated and simple-minded conspiracy theorists pressed me for my opinion about whether abusive secret experiments might still be going on (Moreno, 2001). My response: Although I can't prove a negative, it seems quite unlikely that covert human experiments could continue today. Could I be so confident following the admission of research that stretched, if it did not break, the spirit of an international treaty obligation? Could I be so sure that secret human experiments were not now taking place under the sponsorship of U.S. national security entities?

After the attacks, this story, like so many others, understandably took a back seat to the national emergency. Yet I have wondered whether the outrage that greeted revelations of human experiments conducted without adequate consent and under risky circumstances, especially those sponsored by national security agencies, might have been tempered with the change in certain objective conditions. After all, the original scandals concerning the CIA's MKULTRA program and the army's LSD experiments came in the wake of Vietnam and Watergate. Twenty years later, the human radiation experiments controversy surfaced following a largely (for Americans) bloodless victory in the Persian Gulf and in the context of suspicious sequelae of service in the Gulf that again undermined confidence in our government's concern with its men and women in uniform.

Counterfactuals being what they are, it is impossible to be certain that the public outrage about abusive human experiments involving people in uniform, hospitalized patients, institutionalized children, prisoners, and others would have been lessened had the information not become available when it did. But it is hard to argue that, for example, any new revelations about secret state experiments designed to minimize the effects of a terrorist attack would excite quite the public reaction that they would have before September 11. My confidence in this regard might, of course, be short-lived, depending, as I have said, on the course of the international conflict. Yet at least in the short-term, I do not see how one can draw any other conclusion.

That having been said, what shall we expect if the United States and its allies are indeed engaged in a struggle against terrorism that is years in duration, as the president and other leaders have indicated? Without suggesting that history will simply cycle back to a laissez-faire attitude with respect to covert government activity, it seems unlikely that a great deal of public energy would be expended on the kinds of investigations we have witnessed in the past, at least not with the same intensity. Would the American people today applaud spending tens of millions of dollars investigating cold war human radiation experiments, for example, as was the case in the mid-1990s?

In the early 1970s, scandals about unethical human experiments by civilian organizations and a widespread loss of public sympathy for the military preceded the revelations of the army and CIA chemical weapons research. The country was prepared for outrages when they were discovered. What if, nearly thirty years later, the process were to reverse itself? A new preoccupation with "homeland defense" and a renewed respect for the professionals engaged in these efforts, including the granting of greater legal flexibility for espionage activities, could easily spill over into an enhanced image for civilian institutions whose mission is to protect our national survival. Medical organizations and health-care professionals will play an important role in ameliorating the effects of a chemical or biological attack, and the public health system will be needed to identify an outbreak as well as to organize the response. The esteem in which the medical profession is held, so battered in recent years, could well be improved in the eyes of a jittery public through their identification with these initiatives.

Surely, the tradition of civil libertarianism that has always influenced American political thinking will remain. But the strength of the rights-orientation has waxed and waned, depending partly on perceptions of external threats. As we enter a new political and ideological framework, the recent intense concern about the rights and welfare of human research subjects could be blunted. This could come about not only because the public's attention would be focused mainly on matters of large national interest, with room to concentrate on a relatively small set of domestic problems, but also if continued scientific progress is given greater priority, with increased momentum for the research imperative.

All this is not to assert, of course, that the international and domestic conventions governing ethical human experimentation will be erased or even explicitly disavowed. Rather, the energy and dynamism behind the identification of questionable research practices is likely to lessen if a besieged society views science as an important ally and therefore sees occasional ethical improprieties as lapses in judgment rather than as indicators of a larger crisis of humanism in the pursuit of knowledge.

AUTONOMY AND SOLIDARITY IN CLINICAL ETHICS

Some writers have urged that a "principle of community" be incorporated into the pantheon of bioethical principles, particularly concerning research involving populations in underdeveloped countries. Whatever the merits of this proposal, there can be little argument that a principle of autonomy or self-determination has been virtually the philosophical flagship of modern bioethics. I have been among those who argue that the emergence of this principle in the discussion of physician-patient relations marks a qualitative distinction between traditional medical ethics and modern bioethics (Ahronheim et al., 2000). According to the standard analysis, individual rights in health care can only be trumped by a serious public health concern for which there is an available and effective intervention. The communitarian analysis that has been proposed would privilege public well-being to a far greater degree than the standard view.

Without resorting to communitarianism, it is surely plausible to imagine a future in which the press of recent events has stimulated a reevaluation of a strong autonomy presumption. Without knowing the precise content or result of such a reevaluation, we might simply refer to it as a sentiment of social solidarity. This sentiment might not qualify as a valorized "principle" of biomedical ethics or even appear in bioethics textbooks and journal articles per se. Yet it might be perceptible in the way cases in clinical ethics are analyzed, for example, especially if it is one of those sorts of cases in which an analysis modeled on self-determination has never been all that satisfactory.

To explain my point, I need to note what is obvious to even the casual student of clinical bioethics. In cases of terminally ill "moral strangers"—those who lack capacity and whose prior wishes concerning end-of-life care are unknown to any reasonable degree—certain contortions must be performed in order to make an autonomy-based analysis fit. Thus, we apply a "best interests" or even "reasonable person" test. Yet as many have noted, these are largely fictions intended to reproduce, *per impossibile,* the decisions that we imagine the gravely ill patient would have made himself or herself. The real purpose of these exercises often seems to be to reassure ourselves that we retain a coherent doctrine of autonomy-based medical ethics—and besides, what's the alternative?

Thus, when it is urged that the persistently vegetative patient whose individual wishes are wholly unknown must nonetheless continue to be artificially hydrated and indefinitely provided nutrients, what can our autonomy-based medical ethicist say? That the patient's best interests are being violated? But such people have no interests. That such a condition is an affront to human dignity? There is little agreement about what counts as dignity in these extreme cases. That resources are being wasted? Quite apart from its unpleasant implications, the appeal to resource allocation is not an autonomy-based position.

Among the few prominent ethicists who have argued on behalf of continued artificial feeding in such cases is Daniel Callahan. His appeal to what sounds very much like a social solidarity view has been largely dismissed. Nonetheless, as autonomy has less of a hold on our imaginations, his position might well be up for reassessment. However persuaded we might be that, as the court in *Cruzan* stated, artificial feeding is more like a medical treatment than actual eating, a less individualistic society might feel more qualms about finding autonomy-based reasons to let moral strangers die.

A cultural shift of the kind about which I am speculating in light of the recent catastrophe and the impending "war" on terrorism might also sensitize us to the rationale underlying certain current practices that, again, are not comprehended by the regnant principles or modes of analysis. For instance, experienced clinical ethics consultants are familiar with situations in which a duly authorized healthcare agent is both aware of a terminally patient's wishes not to be sustained indefinitely and in concert with healthcare professionals on the appropriate course. Yet this agent may ask for a reasonable amount of time, say one or two days, to bring the rest of the family along toward acceptance of this conclusion of their loved one's life. In my experience, clinical ethicists would accept temporizing for this purpose, perhaps even in the case of a patient who is dead by neurologic criteria.

Yet what patient-centered criteria, either autonomy or beneficence-based, could contemplate such a position? The most obvious theoretical gambit, reference to the patient's likely wishes in favor of familial harmony, is the usual kind of stretch. Surely, it would be more accurate to acknowledge that what is really going on here is the sense that the death of this patient is an event that affects people other than only the patient. Though this event obviously does not have the significance for the patient that it does for the family, it may still have enormous emotional consequences. The instinct to make this the best death possible for the family as well as for the patient is not grounded in the patient's rights, interests, or even preferences, but rather in a latent sense of the importance of social solidarity in the face of death. Whatever one thinks of communitarianism, this fact about our social sensibilities is hard to deny and at best difficult to capture in standard bioethical theory.

A NEW TURN IN BIOETHICS?

I want to be clear about what I am claiming here and what I am not. I am not asserting that the field of bioethics, either in its theory or practices, will necessarily undergo some sudden and basic shift in light of the September 11 tragedies, any more than constitutional interpretation or legal practices will have to be altered, though they too may be affected. I do not anticipate wholesale abandonment of previous theoretical work in bioethics, including a prominent role for autonomy-oriented analysis. Yet as in the law, there will be ripple effects, especially if the struggle against terrorism is protracted and if Americans in particular are forced to come to terms with a level of risk that seemed only to apply to others. A heightened sense of group vulnerability and patriotic unity has implications for the interpretation of underlying values. One need not be a Marxist to appreciate that even philosophy responds to altered facts on the ground. Indeed, that is how bioethics emerged when it did and why it "saved the life of ethics," as Stephen Toulmin noted years ago (1986).

Again, the effects we shall see are as yet underdetermined. For example, at some point attention will return to such relatively mundane issues as federal policy on the use of embryonic stem cells in research. Will a new societal mood turn toward a more aggressive posture in favor of scientific advancement, perhaps as a reaction to what might be perceived as religious fundamentalism? Or will the turn rather be in the direction of extending respect toward these clumps of cells as precursors of precious human life, its frailty so nauseatingly depicted for us all as the World Trade Center collapsed? Or will the course of future developments in stem cell research be among the social issues that seem unaffected by what has transpired?

It is of course too early to tell, but I am inclined to think that the third possibility, that the recent catastrophe will have no effect at all, is the least likely. Historic crossroads do affect the interpretation and application of moral values, if not their foundations (so far as we can distinguish them), and bioethics is nothing if not the interpretation and application of moral values. Even seemingly arcane and distant matters can fall within the web of change in a society's worldview.

Finally, a prescriptive rather than a speculative note: In at least one respect, our field can and should respond to the terrible events of September 11. Even those of us trained mainly in secular bioethics are familiar with certain basic concepts in Jewish and Christian medical ethics, but we are woefully ignorant of Islamic law. Western scholars in all humanistic disciplines now have an urgent responsibility to familiarize themselves with Islamic teachings and integrate Muslim learning as never before. For all our sakes, legitimate Islamic scholarship must be supported, and non-Muslim thinkers must incorporate it into their work. As well, we should reach out to colleagues in Islamic studies both here and abroad. This is a serious enough lapse in a country where there are more Muslims than there are Episcopalians. For bioethics after the terror, this is a lapse in urgent need of correction.

15

Another Impossible Profession

MORAL FIDUCIARIES

Some years ago an observer called psychoanalysis "the impossible profession": How could anyone hope to see into the psyche of another, apart from the vantage point of one's own? When I committed myself to a career in bioethics and the medical humanities, it struck me that psychoanalysis has some competition for this dubious distinction. Those of us who represent the humanities in the education of health professionals face at best a daunting task. We are expected to be original scholars not only in our own basic disciplines but also in connection with issues in health care. As humanists addressing clinicians and scientists, we are also expected to speak with authority on the economics and politics of health care, the system for allocating resources, the psychology of physician-patient relations, and the culture of medicine, among other diverse topics. Who in their right mind would take this on?

People who relish an intellectual challenge and with no lack of self-esteem, that's who. A thick skin is also no disadvantage. Especially in my early years in bioethics, it was not uncommon for physicians subjected to a talk on medical ethics by their department head to exhibit at best indifference and at worst overt hostility, particularly if the speaker was not a close colleague or even a member of the medical fraternity. Nor do we run the risk of offending the clinicians alone. In one medical school in which I worked, my first on-the-job challenge was not a consultation on a profound end-of-life dilemma but a meeting with the senior basic science faculty. They were convinced that I was hired to be a cop who looked over their shoulders to ensure that no improprieties took place in their labs. I don't think I ever fully disabused them of this suspicion.

Nor do we make things easy for ourselves. The same intellectual and ethical standards we impose on our subject matter are directed at our own conduct, and properly so. Some of the most vigorous disagreements among our members continue to be over exactly what it is we should and shouldn't be doing, especially as "ethicists." Partly the problem lies in the fact that this role is not well defined, yet anyone who purports to be an "ethicist" is asking for close inspection. There is justice in the fact that ours is an increasingly scrutinized profession: considering our relatively small numbers, we wield a wildly disproportionate influence on the public conversation about health care. There is also something paradoxical about taking a public role of speaking with authority about ethics without necessarily being engaged in any specific fiduciary relationships. We are, rather, fiduciaries to the society as a whole. What could be more burdensome and more vague that that?

In the early 1990s I gave a talk to a group of ethics committee members from various hospitals in Buenos Aires. A woman asked me if I didn't think that someone who purported to be an ethicist shouldn't also be ethical in their private life. Her colleagues upbraided her in Spanish even before she finished the question. They knew her agenda: as an observant Roman Catholic, she had often expressed the view that anyone who works in ethics should be morally upright themselves, specifically holding a strong pro-life position. I delivered the standard response, that expertise *about* ethics need not imply expertise *in* ethics, that the former involves knowledge of issues and arguments, but that personal grace (however it is defined) does not necessarily follow from possession of that knowledge.

I'm still comfortable with this answer as far as it goes, which isn't far enough to settle some of the problems that have emerged for the profession of bioethics as it struggles to mature. Two of the problems were wholly predictable (I worried about them before they erupted in my book *Deciding Together,* which is about moral consensus in bioethics) and follow from the professionalization of expertise about moral values. When I served as president of the American Society for Bioethics and Humanities, I had good reason to worry about these problems and what they might mean for the profession.

ETHICIST, HEAL THYSELF

Around 2000, a vigorous debate took place about the appropriate relationship between bioethics and for-profit organizations like drug companies. A few companies had established bioethics advisory boards, especially several high-profile firms working on cutting-edge genetics. Some of the critics charged that this "ethics for hire" was a form of intellectual prostitution. As luck would have it, in the larger world of drug development there was also a controversy about conflict of interest on the part of scientists engaged in research. There were allegations of some improper relationships that gave investigators too much incentive to promote a product in which they had some financial interest. This controversy dovetailed with that about bioethics and private interests.

(Full disclosure: for several years I was on the bioethics advisory board for one for-profit company. I agreed to serve after I was convinced that the leadership was serious about ethics, and in fact, they demonstrated this seriousness on several occasions while I was on the board. My compensation was no greater than I would have earned giving a talk.)

Defenders of a bioethics advisory role in industry made several arguments in response. First, no respectable ethics expert would allow his or her opinion to be bought any more than would an expert in any other field, and to the extent that this is a problem, it's bigger than bioethics. Second, the problems that cause corporate leaders to seek ethics advice are genuine. It's a good thing that they are recognized as such, and if people who think about these things don't weigh in, the advice will come from somewhere else, presumably a less informed source. Third, it's important for bioethics to be engaged in the locus of actual decision making, otherwise it will be limited to taking post facto potshots from the sidelines.

Critics replied that all this may be true, but there's still no argument for financial compensation. Yet why shouldn't individuals with skills involving bioethics be compensated for their effort? Money is the lingua franca of private enterprise. Is there something uniquely corrupting about money changing hands in this context? Because I don't believe there is, I think the same conditions of professional integrity should be applied to bioethics consultation in the private sector as to any other professional activity in that context. To assert otherwise is to suggest some special status for ethics, to engage in the mystification of applied ethics, which does at least as great a disservice to the activity as commercial relationships can do.

In another sense this debate cuts to the question: What kind of career is bioethics, and what kind of activity is it? Is it properly limited to a public intellectual role, or is it also that of a consultant with a set of skills that may be offered in the marketplace? Is bioethics an academic pursuit, or is it that and something more? The answers aren't written in stone, and I'm not sure I can give a normative argument, but I do think I can give an institutional one. Since the invigoration of medical ethics and the bioethical turn in the late 1960s, the whole thrust of the field has been outward. Influence has been sought beyond the seminar room into the courtroom, the committee room, the press room, the hearing room and, most recently, the boardroom. A decision to mark off one of these chambers as forbidden territory is a decision to mark off the field as incompatible with whatever goes on there. That result, arrived at a priori, strikes me as extreme.

Moreover, this result would both overestimate the dangers of bioethics in the boardroom and underestimate its dangers elsewhere. The overestimation has to do with the likelihood that wanton bioethical corruption can long go undetected. Though there is never a guarantee, the organized bioethics community has so far not been shy about scrutinizing its colleague's endeavors. The underestimation has to do with the focus on money as the corrupting influence, even though most intellectuals have other motivations, like professional prestige and institutional advancement. We are largely inured to more subtle compromising situations, like sitting on ethics committees and institutional review boards in our workplaces, conflicts that are much more common but far more rarely discussed than bioethics in the for-profit sector. (I leave aside here the rich question of whether ethicists are supposed to be comfortable with all the sources of their institution's income or the ways they go about attaining it.) But surely our expertise should be available to the institution that pays us, right? The question is the answer.

POLITICS AND POLITICIZATION

Another pothole that accompanies emergence into an influential profession is politicization. Here I want to offer an underutilized distinction: *politics* is the way groups of human beings get things done; *politicization* is the distortion of these normal and useful functions by allowing particular ideologies to run away with the process. Under the former, social problems are subjected to management, not always successfully but generally keeping the problems themselves in focus. Under the latter rubric, the problems become less important than making a point.

Thus, I have no illusions about the fact that politics runs through every activity in the social practice of bioethics, including government advisory committees. The two presidential advisory committees I worked for in the Clinton administration were both dominated by Democrats; twenty-five years ago, the President's Commission on Ethical Problems in Medicine seemed able to agree on a "right to health care" until several Carter commissioners cycled off and were replaced by Reagan appointees. In that case, I'm willing to entertain the possibility that such a declaration doesn't necessarily advance a solution to the underlying problems of healthcare access (though I think it would help).

There does come a tipping point when politics-as-usual (not a bad thing at all, as Aristotle taught), is transformed into politicization. In particular cases, reasonable people can often disagree about when that point has been reached. I was one who believed that the balance had tipped when two members of President George W. Bush's bioethics council were relieved of their positions in spring 2004. Crucial to my judgment was a pattern of appointments to other science advisory committees, a pattern that suggested politicization to me and to the Union of Concerned Scientists, who published their report on this subject just a week before the bioethics council members were not renewed.

Others intimately involved in that process have privately assured me that there were good, nonpolitical, but not publishable reasons that at least one of the members was relieved of membership on the council. But even if one attributes the specific situation to a poor public relations sense on the part of the council's leadership, the event came against a background in which the council had recommended a moratorium on human somatic cell nuclear transfer for biomedical research ("research cloning"). This was a more restrictive position that that taken by virtually all groups in the American scientific community. Even at that, it fell short of the total ban favored by the chairman and a substantial plurality of the members. (It has been alleged that only last-minute maneuvering by the chairman prevented a vote that would have explicitly repudiated a complete ban, yielding instead a majority in favor of a moratorium.) Given that presidential advisory committees are appointed by partisan politicians and science groups are not, I am inclined to view the determinations of one as far less likely to be politicized in the pejorative sense than the other.

At this writing, there is a widespread sense that bioethics has succumbed to the culture wars that occupy many American intellectuals and political junkies—probably a pretty narrow slice of the society, but a noisy one. Bioethics e-mail lists have hosted exchanges that reflect the left-right divide on issues of reproduction, genetics, and end-of-life management; a major bioethics journal felt obliged to editorialize its justification for accepting an analytic commentary with which its editors vigorously disagreed; and a group of neoconservatives have established their own journal with a heavy bioethics emphasis, supported by a right-leaning Washington think tank. Further evidence of the schism is the fact that the co-founder of one of the first bioethics centers has organized closed meetings, in which I have participated, of "liberal" and "conservative" bioethicists, in an attempt to discover common ground.

My initial reaction to the politicization of bioethics (or perhaps the bioethics profession, or both), was sadness that the cherished nonpartisan spirit of bioethical discourse as I had known it since the late 1970s was gone forever. People can forgive, but they can't forget, I thought. But as time has passed, I have come to see that bioethics had largely eluded ideological differences by simply deciding that they wouldn't be allowed in the room. Often that happened, as conservative critics charge, by ensuring that we only talk to our friends, who tend to be academic liberals. More frequently, though, the underlying differences were accepted as irreconcilable, and the implications they held for various issues were not energetically pursued. Collegiality and *politesse* prevailed. This was true of the Baby Doe debate of the 1980s and the assisted suicide debate of the 1990s, in my view. Circumstances changed in bioethics as the country became more polarized, as the human embryonic stem cell and reproductive cloning controversies crystallized the implicit tensions that had long subsisted. As well, a new generation of activist young neoconservatives became interested in the field, but their entrance was via right-wing think tanks rather than the traditional venues of major bioethics graduate programs and research centers.

The new political divide in bioethics thus reflects both the larger philosophical struggle taking place in our public life and the fact that bioethical issues are taken more seriously than ever. Most remarkable is the level of attention the matter has received. Prior to the Bush administration's taking office, I wondered whether I should contact an old college friend who had just become a new Republican senator, to warn him that his friends in the White House were about to face a tough issue about human embryonic stem cell research and that they needed to start talking to some experts. But my natural diffidence prevailed: wouldn't I look foolish trying to tell the new administration that such an arcane subject posed a critical policy question?

As I watched the president's speech to the nation on August 9, 2001, I reassessed my political perspicacity.

PROFESSING BIOETHICS NOW

So include, in the portfolio of the professional bioethicist, preparation to articulate a position on the role of the left-right ideological spectrum in relation to the issues that interest us. If the list of qualifications weren't already long enough, this addition seems at first to take us well beyond the impossible. On this one I am more sanguine, however. Our colleagues in the social sciences have long been obliged to locate themselves ideologically, and they have nonetheless managed to sustain coherent disciplinary cultures even while, for example, free market and government interventionist economists pursue an endless debate. Bioethics embraces and overlaps the social sciences, among its many tributaries, so it is right and proper that, as it matures, the culture of bioethics integrates similar internal tensions. Choosing up sides between conservative and liberal on at least some issues could even turn out to be enriching as well as an inevitable sign of a profession that is growing up.

Acknowledgments

So many people have influenced me over the years on the issues discussed in these writings that I tremble to think of those I will inadvertently exclude. Nonetheless, I must at least express my gratitude to Ron Bayer, Tom Beauchamp, Baruch Brody, Dan Callahan, Art Caplan, Eric Cassell, Jim Childress, Evan Derenzo, Zeke Emanuel, Ruth Faden, Jackie Glover, Chris Grady, Dan Guttman, Alice Herb, Jeff Kahn, Jay Katz, Paul Lombardo, Bob Levine, Glenn McGee, Ruth Macklin, Mary Faith Marshall, Anna Mastroianni, Eric Meslin, Tom Murray, Gail Povar, Adil Shamoo, Harold Shapiro, Jeremy Sugarman, Griff Trotter, Leroy Walters, Paul Wolpe, Laurie Zoloth, and the late John Fletcher and Sandy Leikin.

Students and teachers of bioethics all over the world have reason to be jealous of me for the colleagues I have worked with at the University of Virginia since 1998. There is, as well, no bioethics center staff superior to our administrator, Carrie Gumm, and my assistant, Charlene Kaufman.

Thanks to Robert Sloan and his colleagues at Indiana University Press and to Eric Meslin and Richard Miller for their embrace of this project.

As the family of ideas represented in this book has grown, so has my biological family. Leslye, Jarrett, and Jillian are my constant reminders of why all this matters and also why it doesn't.

Credits

The following are reprinted with permission as needed.

Chapter 1, "Is There an Ethicist in the House?" originally appeared as "Is There a Philosopher in the House?" in *Qualitative Sociology* 20:543–552, 1998.

Chapter 2, "Call Me Doctor? Confessions of a Hospital Philosopher," originally appeared in *Journal of Medical Humanities* 12(4):183–196, Winter 1991.

Chapter 3, "Arguing Euthanasia," originally appeared as "Introduction," in *Arguing Euthanasia: The Controversy Over Mercy Killing, Assisted Suicide and the "Right to Die"* (New York: Touchstone/ Simon & Schuster, 1995; Tokyo: Mita Industries, Ltd., 1997).

Chapter 4, "Bioethics Is a Naturalism," originally appeared in *Pragmatic Bioethics,* ed. G. McGee (Nashville, Tenn.: Vanderbilt University Press, 1999).

Chapter 5, "Ethics Consultation as Moral Engagement," originally appeared in *Bioethics* 5(1):44–56, January 1991.

Chapter 6, "Ethics by Committee: The Moral Authority of Consensus," originally appeared in the *Journal of Medicine and Philosophy* 13:411–432, 1988 (http:/www.tandf.co.uk/journals)

Chapter 7, "Goodbye to All That: The End of Moderate Protectionism in Human Subjects Research," originally appeared in *The Hastings Center Report* 31:9–17, 2001.

Chapter 8, "Convenient and Captive Populations," originally appeared in *Beyond Consent: Seeking Justice in Research,* ed. J. P. Kahn, A. C. Mastroianni, and J. Sugarman (New York: Oxford University Press, 1998).

Chapter 9, "Regulation of Research in the Decisionally Impaired: History and Gaps in the Current Regulatory System," originally appeared in the *Journal of Health Care Law and Policy* (1 J. Health Care L. & Pol'y 1 [1998]).

Chapter 10, "'The Only Feasible Means': The Pentagon's Ambivalent Relationship with the Nuremberg Code," originally appeared in *The Hastings Center Report* 26:11–19, 1996.

Chapter 11, "Reassessing the Influence of the Nuremberg Code on American Medical Ethics," originally appeared in the *Journal of Contemporary Health Law and Policy,* 12:347–360, 1997.

The article, "Cancer, Truth, and Genetics" by Jonathan D. Moreno, Ph.D., originally appearing in the second quarter, 2004 edition of *Oncologistics* magazine; reprinted here with permission from International Oncology Network. All Rights Reserved. Further duplication without permission is prohibited.

Chapter 13, "An Agenda for Neuroethics," originally appeared in *Nature Reviews Neuroscience* 4:149–53, 2003.

Chapter 14, "Bioethics after the Terror," originally appeared in *American Journal of Bioethics* 2:60–64, 2002.

Bibliography

45 *Code of Federal Regulations* 46, subpart C. 1993. "Additional DHHS Protections Pertaining to Biomedical and Behavioral Research Involving Prisoners as Subjects."

Ackerman, T. F. 1987. "The role of an ethicist in health care." In G. R. Anderson and V. A. Glesnes-Anderson, eds., *Health Care Ethics: A Guide for Decision Makers,* pp. 308–20. Rockville, Md.: Aspen Publications.

———. 1989a. "Conceptualizing the role of the ethics consultant: Some theoretical issues." In J. C. Fletcher, N. Quist, and A. R. Jonsen, eds., *Ethics Consultation in Health Care,* pp. 37–53. Ann Arbor, Mich.: Health Administration Press.

———. 1989b. "Moral problems, moral inquiry, and consultation in clinical ethics." In B. Hoffmaster, B. Freedman, and G. Fraser, eds., *Clinical Ethics: Theory and Practice,* pp. 141–60. Clifton, N.J.: Humana Press.

Advisory Committee on Gulf War Veteran's Illnesses. 1996a "Interim Report." Washington, D.C.: U.S. Government Printing Office.

Advisory Committee on Gulf War Veteran's Illnesses. 1996b "Final Report." Washington, D.C.: U.S. Government Printing Office.

Advisory Committee on Human Radiation Experiments (ACHRE). 1996. *The Human Radiation Experiments.* New York: Oxford University Press.

Alexander, S. 1977. "They decide who lives and who dies." In R. Hunt and J. Arras, eds., *Ethical Issues in Modern Medicine.* Palo Alto, Calif.: Mayfield Publishing Co.

American Psychological Association (APA). 1982. *Ethical Principles in the Conduct of Research with Human Participants.* Washington, D.C.: APA.

Annas, George. J. 1992. "The Nuremberg Code in U.S. Courts: Ethics versus expediency." In G. J. Annas and M. A. Grodin, eds., *The Nazi Doctors and the Nuremberg Code.* New York: Oxford University Press.

Annas, George J, and Michael A. Grodin. 1992. *The Nazi Doctors and the Nuremberg Code: Human Rights in Human Experimentation.* New York: Oxford University Press.

Appelbaum, P. S. 1996. "Drug-free research in schizophrenia: An overview of the controversy." *IRB* 18, 1–3.

Ahronheim, J., J. D. Moreno, and C. Zuckerman. 2000. *Ethics in Clinical Practice,* 2nd ed. Gaithersburg, MD: Aspen.

Assistant Secretary for Special Security Programs. 1952. Memorandum from the Assistant Secretary for Special Security Programs to the Secretary of Defense, 25 April 1952.

Atomic Energy Commission. 1950a. Minutes of the Advisory Committee for Biology and Medicine, Atomic Energy Commission, 8–9 September 1950.

Atomic Energy Commission. 1950b. Advisory Committee for Biology and Medicine, AEC, transcript (partial) of meeting, 10 November 1950. ACHRE no. DOE-012795-C-1.

Baldessarini, R. J. 1978. "Chemotherapy." In A. M. Nicolai, ed., *Harvard Guide to Modern Psychiatry.* Cambridge, Mass.: Harvard University Press.

Barrett v. U.S. 660 F.Supp. 1291, 1317 (S.D.N.Y. 1987).

Beauchamp, Thomas, and James Childress. 2001. *Principles of Biomedical Ethics.* 5th ed. New York: Oxford University Press.

Beecher, Henry K. 1959. "Experimentation in man." *Journal of the American Medical Association* 169, 461–78.

———. 1966. "Ethics and clinical research." *New England Journal of Medicine* 274, 1354–60.

———. 1970. "Research and the Individual." In *Research and the Individual: Human Studies* 119, 122–127.

Benjamin, Martin. 1990. *Splitting the Difference: Compromise and Integrity in Ethics and Politics.* Lawrence: University of Kansas Press.

Bonnie, R. 1997. "Research with cognitively impaired subjects." *Archives of General Psychiatry* 5, 373–87.

Boorse, C. 1981. "On the distinction between disease and illness." In A. L. Caplan, H. T. Englhardt and J. J. McCartney, eds., *Concepts of Health and Disease.* Reading, Mass.: Addison-Wesley.

Bosk, Charles. 1979. *Forgive and Remember.* Chicago: University of Chicago Press.

Brody, Baruch A. 1988. *Life and Death Decision Making.* New York: Oxford University Press.

Brown, Phil. 1985. *Transfer of Care: Psychiatric Deinstitutionalization and Its Aftermath.* New York: Routledge.

Brundage, B. M. 1947. "Clearance of technical documents." Major B. M. Brundage, Chief, Medical Division, AEC, to Declassification Section, 19 March 1947. ACHRE no. DOE-113094-B-4.

Burch, R. W. 1974. "Are there moral experts?" *Monist* 58, 646–58.

Caplan, Arthur. 1980. "Ethical engineers need not apply: The state of applied ethics today." *Science, Technology and Human Values* 6, 24–32.

———. 1983. "Can applied ethics be effective in health care and should it strive to be?" *Ethics* 13, 311–19.

Capron, Alexander M. 1997. "Incapacitated research." *Hastings Center Report* 27, 25–27.

Casberg, Melvin A. 1952. "Human Volunteers in Experimental Research." Melvin Casberg, Chairman, AFMPC, to the Secretary of Defense, DOD, 24 December 1952. ACHRE no. NARA-101294-A.

———. 1953. "Digest: Use of human volunteers in experimental research." Melvin A. Casberg, Chairman, AFMPC, to the Secretary of Defense, DOD, 13 January 1953. ACHRE no. DOD-042595-A.

Caspi A., J. McClay, T. E. Moffitt, J. Mill, J. Martin, I. W. Craig, et al. 2002. "Role of genotype in the cycle of violence in maltreated children." *Science* 297, 5582.

Cassidy, James H. 1984. *American Medicine and Statistical Thinking, 1800–1860.* Cambridge, Mass.: Harvard University Press.

Chayet, N. 1976. "Informed consent of the mentally disabled: A failing fiction." *Psychiatric Annals* 6, 82–89.

Chenn, A., and C. A. Walsh. 2002. "Regulation of cerebral cortical size by control of cell cycle exit in neural precursors." *Science* 297, 365–69.

Christakis, N. 1985. "Do medical student research subjects need special protection?" *IRB* 7, 1–4.

Churchland, Patricia Smith. 1989. *Neurophilosophy: Toward a Unified Science of the Mind-Brain.* Cambridge, Mass.: MIT Press.

Clinton, William Jefferson. 1997. Morgan State University Commencement Address, May 18, 1997.

Cohn, V. E. 1976. "Prison test ban opposed." *Washington Post,* 14 March 1976, A7.

Committee on Medical Sciences. 1953. Transcripts of the Meeting of the Committee on Medical Sciences, RDB, DOD, 27 February 1953.

Cranford, R. E., and A. E. Doudera, eds. 1984. *Institutional Ethics Committees and Health Care Decision Making.* Ann Arbor, Mich.: Health Administration Press.

Cruzan v. Director, Missouri Department of Health, 110 S.Ct. 2841. 1990.

Curran, W. J. 1970. "Governmental regulation of the use of human subjects in medical research: The approach of two federal agencies." In P. A. Freund, ed., *Experimentation with Human Subjects,* pp. 402–54. New York: George Braziller.

Damasio, Antonio. 1994 *Descartes' Error: Emotion, Reason, and the Human Brain.* New York: HarperCollins.

Daniels, N. 1979. "Wide reflective equilibrium and theory acceptance in ethics." *Journal of Philosophy* 76, 256–82.

Department of Defense. 1950a. Transcript of the Meeting of the Committee on Medical Sciences of the Research and Development Board, 31 January–1 February 1950, pp. 61–66.

Department of Defense. 1950b. Transcript of the Meeting of the Committee on Medical Sciences of the Research and Development Board, 23 May 1950.

Department of Defense. 1951. Annual Report of the Armed Forces Medical Policy Council, Department of Defense, to the Secretary of Defense, 30 June 1951.

Department of Defense. 1952a. Minutes of a meeting from the Department of Defense service representatives, 11 February 1952.

Department of Defense. 1952b. Transcript of the Meeting of the Committee on Chemical Warfare, RDB, DOD, 10 November 1952, p. 128. ACHRE no. NARA-1025.

Dewey, John. 1935. *Liberalism and Social Action.* New York: Capricorn.

———. 1958. *Experience and Nature.* New York: Dover.

———. [1929] 1960. *The Quest for Certainty: A Study of the Relation of Knowledge and Action.* New York: Putnam.

———. 1971. *Reconstruction of Philosophy.* Boston: Beacon Press.

Donagan, Alan. 1977. "Informed consent in therapy and experimentation." *Journal of Medicine and Philosophy* 2, 318–29.

Downey, T. J. 1975. "Report on human experimentation conducted or funded by the U.S. Army." *Congressional Record* 121, 27934.

Dresser, R. 1996. "Mentally disabled research subjects: The enduring policy issues." *Journal of the American Medical Association* 276, 67.

Dresser, R., and P. Whitehouse. 1997. "Emergency research and research involving subjects with cognitive impairment: Ethical connections and contrasts." *Journal of the American Geriatric Society* 45, 521.

Duff, R. S., and A. G. M. Campbell 1973. "Moral and ethical dilemmas in the special care nursery." *New England Journal of Medicine* 289, 890–94.

Editorial. 2002. "In search of language genes." *Nature Neuroscience* 4, 1049.

Englehardt, H. Tristram, Jr. 1986. *The Foundations of Bioethics.* New York: Oxford University Press.

Ethridge, Elizabeth W. 1972. *The Butterfly Caste: A Social History of Pellagra in the South.* Westport, Conn.: Greenwood Publishing Company.

Exec. Order no. 12,975, 60 Red. Reg. 52,063. 1995.

Faden, Ruth L., and Tom L. Beauchamp. 1986. *A History and Theory of Informed Consent.* New York: Oxford University Press.

Faden, Ruth L., et al. 1996. "U.S. medical researchers, the Nuremberg doctor trial and the Nuremberg Code: A review of the findings of the Advisory Committee on Human Radiation Experiments." *Journal of the American Medical Association* 276, 1667.

Federal Food Drug and Cosmetic Act. 21 U.S.C. ss 355. 1997.

Federal Food Drug and Cosmetic Act Amendments. 21 U.S.C. ss 355(i). 1997.

Federal Policy for the Protection of Human Subjects; Notices and Rules. 56 Fed. Reg. 28002-28032 (June 18, 1991).

Fletcher, Joseph F. 1966. *Situation Ethics.* Philadelphia: Westminster Press.

Foot, P. 1967. "Introduction." In P. Foot, ed., *Theories of Ethics,* pp. 1–15. New York: Oxford University Press.

Fost, N., and R. E. Cranford. 1985. "Hospital ethics committees: Administrative aspects." *Journal of the American Medical Association* 253, 2687–92.

Fox, Renee C. 1974. *Experiment Perilous: Physicians and Patients Facing the Unknown.* Philadelphia: University of Pennsylvania Press.

Gardella, J. W. 1953. "Criticisms of Principles, Policies and Rules of the Surgeon General, Department of the Army, relating to the use of Human Volunteers in Medical Research Contracts awarded by the Army." Memorandum to "GPB" [Harvard Medical School Dean Berry] from "JWG" [Assistant Dean Gardella]. ACHRE no. IND-072595-A.

Germany (Territory under Allied occupation, 1945–1955: U.S. Zone). *Trials of War Criminals before the Nuernberg Military Tribunals under Control Council Law no. 10, Nuernberg, October 1946–April 1949.* Vol. 2. Washington, D.C.: Government Printing Office.

Glantz, Leonard H. 1992. "The influence of the Nuremberg Code on U.S. statutes and regulations." In G. J. Annas and M. A. Grodin, eds., *The Nazi Doctors and the Nuremberg Code.* New York: Oxford University Press.

———. 1994. "The Law of Experimentation with Children," in M. A. Grodin and L. A. Glantz, *Children as Research Subjects: Science, Ethics and Law.* New York: Oxford University Press.

Golby, A. J., J. D. E. Gabrieli, J. Y. Chiao, and J. L. Eberhardt. 2001. "Differential responses in the fusiform region to same-race and other-race faces." *Nature Neuroscience* 4, 845–50.

Grob, Gerald N. 1994. *The Mad among Us: A History of the Care of America's Mentally Ill.* New York: Free Press.

Grodin, M. A. 1992. "Historical origins of the Nuremberg Code." In G. J. Annas and M. A. Grodin, eds., *The Nazi Doctors and the Nuremberg Code: Human Rights and Human Experimentation.* New York: Oxford Press.

Harkness, J. E. 1996. "Research behind Bars: A History of Nontherapeutic

Research on American Prisoners." Ph.D. diss., University of Wisconsin Department of History.

High, D. M., et al. 1994. "Guidelines for addressing ethical and legal issues in Alzheimer disease research: A position paper." *Alzheimer Disease and Associated Disorders* 8 (Suppl. 4), 66–74.

Hoffman, D., and J. Schwartz. 1998. "Proxy consent to participation of the decisionally impaired in medical research: Maryland's policy initiative." *Journal of Health Care Law & Policy* 1, 136.

Humphry, Derek. 2002. *Final Exit.* 3rd ed. New York: Dell Publishing.

Humphreys, L. 1970. *Tearoom Trade: Impersonal Sex in Public Places.* Chicago: Adeline Publishing Co.

In the Matter of Quinlan, 70 N.J. 10, 355 A.2d 647, *cert. Denied,* 429 U.S. 922. 1976.

"It's over Debbie." *Journal of the American Medical Association* 259, 2094. 1988.

Jackson, Stephen S. 1952a. Stephen S. Jackson, Assistant General Counsel in the Office of the Secretary of Defense and Counsel for the Armed Forces Medical Policy Council, DOD, to Melvin A. Casberg, Chairman of the Armed Forces Medical Policy Council, 13 October 1952. ACHRE no. NARA-101294-A.

———. 1952b. Stephen S. Jackson, Assistant General Counsel in the Office of the Secretary of Defense and Counsel for the Armed Forces Medical Policy Council, DOD, to Melvin A. Casberg, Chairman of the Armed Forces Medical Policy Council, 22 October 1952. ACHRE no. NARA-101294-A.

Jacoby, Russell. 1987. *The Last Intellectuals: American Culture in the Age of Academe.* New York: Basic Books.

James, William. 1890. *The Principles of Psychology.* New York: Henry Holt.

———. 1968. "On a certain blindness in human beings." In J. J. McDermott, ed., *The Writings of William James,* 629–45. New York: Modern Library.

Jonas, Hans. 1970. "Philosophical reflections on experimenting with human subjects." In P. A. Freund, ed., *Experimentation with Human Subjects.* New York: George Braziller.

———. 1972. *Experimentation with Human Beings.* Ed. J. Katz. New York: Russell Sage Foundation.

Jonsen, A. R. 1986. "Casuistry and clinical ethics." *Theoretical Medicine* 7, 65–74.

Jonsen, A. R., and Stephen Toulmin. 1988. *The Abuse of Casuistry.* Berkeley: University of California Press.

Kamm, F. M. 1988. "Ethics, applied ethics, and applying applied ethics." In D. M. Rosenthal and F. Shehadi, eds., *Applied Ethics and Ethical Theory,* pp. 162–87. Salt Lake City: University of Utah Press.

Karlawish, J. H. T., and G. A. Sachs. 1997. "Research on the cognitively impaired: Lessons and warnings from the emergency research debate." *Journal of the American Geriatric Society* 45, 475.

Katz, Jay., et al. 1972. *Experimentation with Human Beings: The Authority of the Investigator, Subject, Professions, and State in the Human Experimentation Process.* New York: Russell Sage Foundation.

———. 1991. "The consent principle of the Nuremberg Code: Its significance then and now." In *The Nazi Doctors and the Nuremberg Code,* ed. G. J. Annas and M. A. Grodin, p. 228. New York: Oxford University Press.

Keyserlingk, E. W., et al. 1995. "Proposed guidelines for the participation of persons with dementia as research subjects." *Perspectives in Biology and Medicine* 38, 319–62.

Kliegman, R. M., M. B. Mahowad, and S. J. Younger. 1986. "In our best interests: Experience and workings of an ethic review committee." *Journal of Pediatrics* 188, 178–88.

Knoppers, B. M., and S. LeBris. 1991. "Recent advances in medically assisted conception: Legal, ethical and social issues." *American Journal of Law and Medicine* 17, 335.

Kopelman, L. 1993. "Cynicism among medical students." *Journal of the American Medical Association* 250, 2006–10.

Koritz, T. 1953. "I was a human guinea pig." *Saturday Evening Post,* 25 July 1953, 27, 79–80.

Koski, Greg. 1999. "Resolving Beecher's Paradox." *Accountability in Research* 7, 1999.

Krikorian, Yervant H. 1944. *Naturalism and the Human Spirit.* New York: Columbia University Press.

Krugman, S. 1986. "The Willowbrook hepatitis studies revisited: Ethical aspects." *Reviews of Infectious Diseases* 8, 157–62.

Lalor, W. G. 1952. "Security measures on chemical warfare and biological warfare." W. G. Lalor, Secretary, Joint Chiefs of Staff, to Chief of Staff, U.S. Army, Chief of Naval Operations, Chief of Staff, U.S. Air Force, 3 September 1952. ACHRE no. NARA-012495-A.

Lasagna, Louis 1971. "Some ethical problems in clinical investigation." In E. Mendehlsohn, J. P. Swazey, and H. Taviss, eds., *Human Aspects of Biomedical Innovation.* Cambridge, Mass.: Harvard University Press.

———. 1977. "Prisoner subjects and drug testing." *Federation Proceedings* 36, 2349.

———. 1994. "Louis Lasagna interview by Jon M. Harkness and Suzanne White-Junod (ACHRE), transcript of audio recording, 13 December 1994." ACHRE Research Project Series, Interview Program File, Ethics Oral History Project, 5.

Lasagna, L. M., and J. M. Von Felsinger. 1972. "The Volunteer Subject in

Research." In J. Katz, ed., *Experimentation with Human Beings,* pp. 623–24. New York: Russell Sage Foundation.

Lederer, Susan E. 1995. *Subjected to Science: Experimentation in America before the Second World War.* Baltimore: Johns Hopkins University Press.

Lederer, Susan E., and Michael A. Grodin. 1994. "Historical overview: Pediatric experimentation." In M. A. Grodin and L. H. Glantz, eds., *Children as Research Subjects: Science, Ethics, and Law.* New York: Oxford University Press.

Levine, C. 1984. "Questions and (some very tentative) answers about hospital ethics committees." *Hastings Center Report* 14, 9–12.

———. 1989. "Military medical research: Are there ethical exceptions?" *IRB* 11, 5–7.

Levine, R. 1997. "Proposed regulations for research involving those institutionalized as mentally infirm: A consideration of their relevance in 1996." *IRB* 18, 1.

Levy, B. J., and M. C. Anderson. 2002. "Inhibitory processes and the control of memory retrieval." *Trends in Cognitive Science* 6, 299–305.

Lieberman, J. A., S. Stroup, E. Laska, et al. 1999. "Issues in clinical research design: Principles, practices, and controversies." In H. A. Pincus, J. A. Lieberman, and S. Ferris, eds., *Ethics in Psychiatric Research,* pp. 25–26. Washington, D.C.: American Psychiatric Association.

Lo, B. 1987. "Behind closed doors: Promises and pitfalls of ethics committees." *New England Journal of Medicine* 317, 46–49.

Lynn, J. 1984. "Roles and functions of institutional ethics committees: The President's Commission's view." In R. E. Cranford and A. E. Doudera, eds., *Institutional Ethics Committees and Health Care Decision Making,* pp. 22–30. Ann Arbor, Mich.: Health Administration Press.

MacIntyre, Alasdair. 1981. *After Virtue.* Notre Dame, Ind.: University of Notre Dame Press.

Macklin, R. 1988 "The inner workings of an ethics committee." *Hastings Center Report* 18, 15–20.

Marineau, Rene F. 1989. *Jacob Levy Moreno, 1889–1974: Father of Psychodrama, Sociometry, and Group Psychotherapy.* New York: Routledge.

McConnell, T. E. 1984. "Objectivity and moral expertise." *Canadian Journal of Philosophy* 14, 193–216.

McDermott, Walsh. 1967. "Opening comments on the changing mores of biomedical research." *Annals of Internal Medicine* 67 (Suppl. 7), 39–42.

Milgram, Stanley. 1974. *Obedience to Authority.* New York: Harper & Row.

Mill, J. S. 1975. "Of the limits of the authority of society over the individual." In D. Spitz, ed., *On Liberty,* pp. 70–86. New York: W.W. Norton.

Mitford, Jessica. 1973. "Experiments behind bars: Doctors, drug companies, and prisoners." *Atlantic Monthly* 23, 64–73.

More, Thomas. 1997 [1516]. *Utopia.* Boston: Bedford/St. Martin's.

Moreno, John D. 1981. "The continuity of madness: Pragmatic naturalism and mental health in America." In Arthur Caplan et al., eds., *Concepts of Health and Disease: Interdisciplinary Perspectives.* San Diego, Calif.: Pearson Addison Wesley.

———. 1988. "Ethics by committee: The moral authority of consensus." *Journal of Medicine and Philosophy* 13, 411–32.

———. 1991. "Clinical ethics as moral engagement." *Bioethics* 5, 44–56.

———. 1995. *Deciding Together: Bioethics and Moral Consensus.* New York: Oxford University Press.

———. 1996a. "Do bioethics commissions hijack public debate?" *Hastings Center Report* 26, 46.

———. 1996b. "Ethical considerations of industry-sponsored research: The use of human subjects." *Journal of the American College of Nutrition* 15, 35s.

———. 1996c. "The only feasible means: The Pentagon's ambivalent relationship with the Nuremberg Code." *Hastings Center Report* 26, 11.

———. 1997. "Reassessing the influence of the Nuremberg Code in American medical ethics." *Journal of Contemporary Health Law & Policy* 13, 347.

———. 1998. "Regulation of research in the decisionally impaired: History and gaps in the current regulatory system." *Journal of Health Care Law and Policy* 1, 1–21.

———. 1999. *Undue Risk: Secret State Experiments on Humans.* New York: W. H. Freeman.

Moreno, J. D., and S. Lederer. 1996. "Revising the history of the cold war research ethics." *Kennedy Institute of Ethics Journal* 6, 223.

Moreno, J. L. 1987a. "The autobiography of J. L. Moreno, M.D."

———. 1987b. "The autobiography of J. L. Moreno, M.D.—abridged." *Journal of Group Psychotherapy, Psychodrama & Sociometry.*

Murray, Thomas. 1987. "Medical ethics, moral philosophy and moral tradition." *Social Science and Medicine* 25, 637–44.

Mussells, F. Lloyd. 1952. "Human experimentation." F. Lloyd Mussells, Executive Director, Committee on Medical Sciences, RDB, DOD, to Floyd L. Miller, Vice Chairman, Research and Development Board, DOD, 12 November 1952. ACHRE no. NARA-071194-A-2.

National Bioethics Advisory Commission. 1997. Full Commission Meeting. Arlington, Virginia, May 17, 1997.

National Bioethics Advisory Commission. 1998. *Research Involving Persons with Mental Disorders That May Affect Decision Making Capacity.* Washington, D.C.: U.S. Government Printing Office.

National Bioethics Advisory Committee. 1996. Meeting of the National Bioethics Advisory Committee, October 4.

National Commission for the Protection of Human Subjects of Biomedical Research. 1976. *Research Involving Prisoners: Appendix to Report and Recommendations.* Washington, D.C.: U.S. Department of Health, Education and Welfare.

National Commission for the Protection of Human Subjects of Biomedical and Behavioral Research. 1978. *National Commission for the Protection of Human Subjects of Biomedical and Behavioral Research, Report and Recommendations: Research Involving Those Institutionalized as Mentally Infirm.* DHEW Pub. no. (OS) 78-0006, 1978.

National Commission for the Protection of Human Subjects of Biomedical and Behavioral Research. 1979. *The Belmont Report: Ethical Principles and Guidelines for the Protection of Human Subjects.* Federal Register Document 79-12065, April 18, 1979.

"New York seeks to tighten rules on medical research." *New York Times,* 27 September 1996, B4.

Nickel, J. W. 1988. "Philosophy and policy." In D. M. Rosenthal and F. Shehadi, eds., *Applied Ethics and Ethical Theory,* pp. 139–48. Salt Lake City: University of Utah Press.

Nietzsche, Friedrich. 1995 [1891]. *Thus Spake Zarathustra.* New York: Dover.

Novack, D. H. 1979. "Changes in physicians' attitudes toward telling the cancer patient." *Journal of the American Medical Association* 241, 897–900.

Nussbaum, Martha C. 1994. *The Therapy of Desire.* Princeton, N.J.: Princeton University Press.

Office for Protection from Research Risks Division of Human Subject Protection. 1994. *Evaluation of Human Subject Protections in Schizophrenia Research Conducted by the University of California, Los Angeles.* New York: Office for Protection from Research Risks.

Office of the Secretary of Defense. 1950. Memorandum from the Assistant Secretary of the Army to the Director of Medical Services, Office of the Secretary of Defense, 3 May 1950.

O'Hara, J. L. 1953. "The most unforgettable character I've met." *Reader's Digest,* May 1948, 30–35.

Oken, D. 1961. "What to tell cancer patients: A study of medical attitudes." *Journal of the American Medical Association* 175, 1120–28.

Olaussen, H., Y. Lamarre, H. Backlund, C. Morin, B. G. Wallin, G. Starck, et al. 2002. "Unmyelinated tactile afferents signal touch and project to insular cortex." *Nature Neuroscience* 5, 900–904.

Pappworth, Maurice Henry. 1967. *Human Guinea Pigs: Experimentation on Man.* Boston: Beacon Press.

Peirce, C. S. 1955. "How to make our ideas clear." In J. Buchler, ed., *Philosophical Writings of Pierce.* New York: Dover.

Potler, C., V. L. Sharp, and S. Remnick. 1994. "Prisoners' access to HIV experimental trials: Legal, ethical, and practical considerations." *Journal of Acquired Immune Deficiency Syndrome* 7, 1086–1094.

President's Commission for the Study of Ethical Problems in Medicine and Biomedical and Behavioral Research. 1982. *Compensating for Research Injuries: The Ethical and Legal Implications of Programs to Redress Injured Subjects.* Vol. I: *Report.* Washington, D.C.: U.S. Government Printing Office.

President's Commission for the Study of Ethical Problems in Medicine and Biomedical and Behavioral Research. 1983a. *Deciding to Forgo Life-Sustaining Treatment.* Washington, D.C.: U.S. Government Printing Office.

President's Commission for the Study of Ethical Problems in Medicine and Biomedical and Behavioral Research. 1983b *Implementing Human Subject Regulations.* Washington, D.C.: U.S. Government Printing Office.

"Prison research: Ethics behind bars." *Nature* 242, 153. 1973.

Proctor, Robert N. 1992. "Nazi doctors, racial medicine, and human experimentation." In G. J. Annas and M. A. Grodin, eds., *The Nazi Doctors and the Nuremberg Code: Human Rights and Human Experimentation.* New York: Oxford University Press.

Protection of Human Subjects. 43 Fed. Reg. 11,328, 11,330, 11,332 (1978).

Protection of Human Subjects. 56 Fed. Reg. 28,002 (1991).

Protection of Human Subjects. 45 CFR ss 46.101–.404 (1991).

Protection of Human Subjects. 45 CFR ss 46.101–.409 (1997).

Quill, T. 1991. "Death and dignity: A case of individualized decision making." *New England Journal of Medicine* 324, 691–694.

Quine, W. V. O. 1960. *Word and Object.* Cambridge, Mass.: MIT Press.

Rachels, James. 1986. *The End of Life.* New York: Oxford University Press.

Radbill, S. X. (1979) "The use of children in pediatric research." Paper delivered at American Association for the History of Medicine, Pittsburgh, May 4, 1979.

Railton, P. 1986. "Moral realism." *Philosophical Review* 95, 163–207.

Ramsey, Paul. 1970. *The Patient as Person: Explorations in Medical Ethics.* New Haven, Conn.: Yale University Press.

Rapalski, Adam J. 1953. "The attached letter I believe is self-explanatory." Adam J. Rapalski, Administrator, Armed Forces Epidemiological Board, DOD, to Collin McLeod, President, Armed Forces Epidemiological Board, DOD, 2 March 1953. ACHRE no. NARA-012395-A-5.

Redman, Leslie M. 1951. Leslie M. Redman, Los Alamos Laboratory, to Dr. Alberto F. Thompson, Chief, Technical Information Service, DBM, 22 January 1951. ACHRE no. DOE-051094-A-609.

Refshauge, W. 1977. "The place for international standards in conducting research for humans." *Bulletin of the World Health Organization* 55, 133–

35 (Suppl. 1977) (quoting H. K. Beecher, "Research and the individual," *Human Studies* 279 [1970]).

Reisman, John S. 1965 "Resolution of the Council." Dr. John S. Reisman, the Executive Secretary, NAHC, to Dr. James A. Shannon, 6 December 1965.

Report on the National Conference on the Legal Environment of Medicine. 1959. 27–28 May 1959. Chicago: National Society for Medical Research.

Rilling, J. K., D. A. Gutman, T. R. Zeh, G. Pagnoni, G. S. Berns, and C. D. Kilts. 2002. "A neural basis for social cooperation." *Neuron* 35, 395–405.

Robertson, J. A. 1984. "Ethics committees in hospitals: Alternative structures and responsibilities." *Connecticut Medicine* 48, 441–44.

Rollins, Betty. 1998. *Last Wish.* New York: Public Affairs.

Rorty, Richard 1961. "Pragmatism, categories, and language." *Philosophical Review* 70, 197–223.

———. 1979. *Philosophy and the Mirror of Nature.* Princeton, N.J.: Princeton University Press.

———. 1983. "Method and morality." In N. Hann, ed., *Social Science and Moral Inquiry,* pp. 155–76. New York: Columbia University Press.

Rosenthal, Sandra B. 1990. *Speculative Pragmatism.* Peru, Ill.: Open Court Publishing Co.

———. 1996. "Classical American pragmatism: The other naturalism." *Metaphilosophy* 27, 399.

Rothman, David J. 1994. *Strangers at the Bedside: A History of How Law and Bioethics Transformed Medical Decision Making.* New York: Basic Books.

Ryder, John, ed. 1994. *American Philosophic Naturalism.* Amherst, N.Y.: Prometheus Books.

Satcher, David. 1997. "Statement of David Satcher, M.D., Ph.D., Director, CDC." HHS Oversight Biomedical Ethics: Hearing Before the Subcommittee on Human Resources of the House Committee on Government Reform and Oversight, 105th Cong., 1997 WL 10570903.

Schacter, Daniel L. 2001. *The Seven Sins of Memory: How the Mind Forgets and Remembers.* Boston: Houghton Mifflin.

Schwartz, J. 1998. "Office of the Md. Att'y Gen., Second Report of the Attorney General's Working Group." App at A-9, in *Journal of Healthcare Law and Policy* 1, 279–81.

Secretary of Defense. 1951. "Directive."' 21 December 1951. Record Group 220 (Presidential Committees, Commissions, and Boards) at the National Archives and Records Administration, Washington, D.C.

Secretary of Defense. 1953. "Use of human volunteers in experimental research." Secretary of Defense to the Secretary of the Army, Secretary of the Navy, Secretary of the Air Force, 26 February 1953. ACHRE no. DOD-082394-A.

Shamoo, A. E., and T. J. Keay. 1996. "Ethical concerns about relapse studies." *Cambridge Quarterly of Healthcare Ethics* 5, 373–86.

Siegler, M. 1986. "Ethics committees: Decisions by bureaucracy." *Hastings Center Report* 16, 22–24.

Simmel, Georg 1950. "Superordination and subordination." In K. Wolff, ed., *The Sociology of Georg Simmel.* Glencoe, Ill.: Free Press.

Singer, Peter (1972) "Moral experts." *Analysis* 32, 115–17.

———. 1982. "How do we decide?" *Hastings Center Report* 12, 9–11.

Stanley, Douglas. 1978. *The Technological Conscience.* New York: Free Press.

Still, G. F. 1965. *The History of Pediatrics.* London: Dawsons of Pall Mall.

Stone, Robert S. 1950. "Irradiation of human subjects as a medical experiment." Paper presented to Department of Defense, NEPA Medical Advisory Committee on 31 January 1950. ACHRE no. NARA 070794-A.

"Supplemental report of the judicial council." 1946. Proceedings of the House of Delegates Annual Meeting, 9–11 December 1946. *Journal of the American Medical Association* 132, 1090.

Task Force on Human Subject Research. 1994. "A Report on the Use of Radioactive Materials in Human Subjects Research that Involved Residents of State-Operated Facilities within the Commonwealth of Massachusetts from 1943–1973." ACHRE no. MASS-072194-A.

T.D. v. N.Y. State Office of Mental Health. A.D.2d, 650 N.Y.S.2d 173 (1st Dept. 1996).

T.D. v. New York State Office of Mental Health. 1996. 60 N.Y.S.2d 173 (N.Y. App. Div. 1996).

T.D. v. New York State Office of Mental Health. 1997. 60 N.Y.S.2d 173 (N.Y. App. Div. 1996), appeal dismissed by 680 N.E.2d. (N.Y. 1997).

T.D. v. New York State Office of Mental Health. 1996. 60 N.Y.S.2d 173 (N.Y. App. Div. 1996) leave to appeal granted by 684 N.E.2d (N.Y. 1997).

T.D. v. New York State Office of Mental Health. 1996. 60 N.Y.S.2d 173 (N.Y. App. Div. 1996) appeal dismissed by 1997 WL 785461 (N.Y. Dec. 22, 1997).

Toulmin, Stephen E. 1986. "How medicine saved the life of ethics." In Joseph. P. Demarco and Richard M. Fox, eds., *New Directions in Ethics.* New York: Routledge and Kegan Paul.

Trout, M. E. 1974. "Should research in prisons be barred?" *Journal of Legal Medicine* 2, 2.

Underwood, George V. 1953a. George V. Underwood, Director of the Executive Office of the Secretary of Defense, to Deputy Secretary Foster, 4 January 1953.

———. 1953b. "Use of human volunteers in experimental research." George V. Underwood, Director, Executive Office, Office of the Secretary of Defense to Mr. Keyes, Deputy Secretary of Defense, 5 February 1953. ACHRE no. DOD-062194-A.

United States v. Karl Brandt et al. 1949. In *The Medical Case: Trials of War Criminals before the Nuremberg Medical Tribunals under Control Council Law No. 10.* Washington, D.C.: U.S. Government Printing Office.

United States v. Stanley, 483 U.S. 669. 1987.

United States Department of Energy, Office of Health and Environmental Research. 1993. *Human Subjects Research Handbook Second Edition: Appendix—The Nuremberg Code.* Washington, D.C.: United States Government Printing Office.

United States General Accounting Office. 1996. *U.S. Gen Acct. Off., Report to the Ranking Minority Member, Committee on Governmental Affairs, U.S. Senate, Scientific Research: Continued Vigilance Critical to Protecting Human Subjects,* GAO/HEHS Doc. No. 96-72 (1996).

United States Government Human Radiation Interagency Working Group. 1997. *Building Public Trust: Actions to Respond to the Report of the Advisory Committee on Human Radiation Experiments.* Washington, D.C.: U.S. Government Printing Office.

United States House of Representatives Subcommittee on Government Operations. Hearings on Informed Consent, May 8, 1997.

Unknown author to the Advisory Board on Biology and Medicine. 8 October 1947. ACHRE no. DOE-0151094-A-502.

"U.S. seeks duplicate of Russian anthrax microbe to be used to check vaccine." *Washington Post,* 5 September 2001, A16.

Veatch, Robert M. 1983. "Definitions of life and death: Should there be consistency?" In M. W. Shaw and A. E. Doudera, eds., *Defining Human Life: Medical, Legal and Ethical Implications.* Ann Arbor, Mich.: AUPHA Press.

Wasson, T., and G. H. Brieger. 1987. "Von Jauregg, J. W." In *Nobel Prize Winners: An H .W. Wilson Biographical Dictionary,* 1092-93. New York: H. W. Wilson Co.

Weir, R. F. 1987. "Pediatric ethics committees: Ethical advisors or legal watchdogs?" *Law, Medicine and Health Care* 15, 99–109.

Whittemore, G. 1988. "A Crystal Ball in the Shadows of Nuremberg and Hiroshima: The Ethical Debate over Human Experimentation to Develop a Nuclear Powered Bomber, 1946–1951." In *Science, Technology and the Military,* ed. E. Mendelsohn, M. R. Smith, and P. Weingart. Dordrecht: Kluwer Academic Publishers, 1988.

Wilson, Carroll L. 1947a. Carroll L. Wilson, General Manager of the AEC, to Stafford Warren, University of California at Los Angeles, 30 April 1947. ACHRE no. DOE-052094-A-439.

———. 1947b. Carroll L. Wilson, General Manager of the AEC, to Robert Stone, University of California, 5 November 1947. ACHRE no. DOE-052295-A-1.

Winston; J. S., B. A. Strange, J. Doherty, and R. J. Dolan. 2002. *Nature Neuroscience* 5, 277–83.

World Medical Association. 1964. Declaration of Helsinki: Recommendations Guiding Medical Doctors in Biomedical Research Involving Human Subjects, adopted by the Eighteenth World Medical Assembly, Helsinki, Finland.

Worthley, H. N. 1952. "Use of volunteers in experimental research." H. N. Worthley, Executive Director, Committee on Chemical Warfare, RDB, DOD, to the Director of Administration, Office of the Secretary of Defense, 9 December 1952. ACHRE no. NARA-101294-A.

Index

JONATHAN D. MORENO is Kornfeld Professor and Director of the Center for Biomedical Ethics at the University of Virginia and a fellow of the Center for American Progress. He is also a fellow of the Hastings Center and the New York Academy of Medicine, and a faculty affiliate of the Kennedy Institute of Ethics at Georgetown University. He has been a senior staff member for two presidential commissions and an advisor to the White House Office of Science and Technology Policy, the National Institutes of Health, the Department of Health and Human Services, the National Academy of Sciences, and the Howard Hughes Medical Institute. He is past president of the American Society for Bioethics and Humanities.